THE 5 HUNGERS

THE 5 HUNGERS

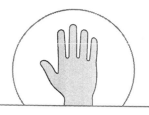

STEALTH APPETITES YOU CAN SATISFY
WITHOUT OVEREATING

BEVERLY HYATT NEVILLE, PHD, RD

BookWise Publishing
www.bookwisepublishing.com

Book design: Eden Design, Salt Lake City, Utah
ISBN for trade paperback: 9781477561539

First Printing

Visit the publisher's website:
http://www.letmereadit.com

To all my students

"We are indeed much more than what we eat, but what we eat can nevertheless help us to be much more than what we are."

— ADELLE DAVIS —

CONTENTS

THE HANDMAID OF GENIUS

Part I: THE THUMB
THE FIRST HUNGER IS FOR SUGAR

Part II: THE INDEX FINGER
THE SECOND HUNGER IS PHYSICAL EMPTINESS

Part III: THE MIDDLE FINGER
THE THIRD HUNGER IS EMOTIONAL EMPTINESS

Part IV: THE RING FINGER
THE FOURTH HUNGER IS FOR STABILITY

"I cannot count the good people I know who to my mind would be even better if they bent their spirits to the study of their own hungers."

— M. F. K. FISHER —

THE HANDMAID OF GENIUS

✣ 1 ✣

Why Five?

MARK TWAIN TRAVELED through Europe in the 1870s, staying in luxury hotels with reputations for the best cuisine in the world. However, in 1879 he wrote that he was longing for good old American food.[1] He made a list of the meals he was most hungry for, mentioning foods from his childhood in Hannibal, Missouri and places he had visited in America.

Notable on his list were lake trout, radishes, turkey, cranberry sauce and apple pie. The meal he fantasized about grew to eighty items before he was done.

Good food and appetites were important to Twain, a noted observer of human nature. He later wrote *"Hunger is the handmaid of genius."*[2] While he may have meant it as a metaphor—like saying necessity is the mother of invention—when we think about hunger or deciding what to eat, *genius* is hardly the first term that comes to mind. Quite the opposite, according to national health statistics.

And yet, we can each become a genius regarding hunger once we realize there are only five hungers to keep track of.

---

1. Twain, M. (1880) *A Tramp Abroad,* available at Project Gutenberg
2. Twain, M., (1897) *Following the Equator: A Journey around the World,* Chapter 43, American Publishing Co., Hartford, CT

Why five, you ask?

The simple answer: five is a number we can remember.

After decades of researching, teaching, and working in the fields of public health and nutrition, I'm convinced we've made the subject of food too complex and confusing. Who can remember anything from the fog of ideas we've read, seen on television, or discussed with co-workers and friends?

Magazines in check-out stands offer the perfect recipes for the perfect diets for the perfect bodies. The list of the top-selling 100 books on Amazon always includes fifteen to twenty new food-related titles. As I write this, six of the top ten titles on the *New York Times Hardcover Advice, How-To, and Miscellaneous* category involve food. I'm sure you've read many of the books I reference in the Appendix; in fact, if this is the first food, diet, nutrition, or health book you've ever read, you are in a small minority.

To make it worse, every day a new nutritional study is released. A celebrity endorses a new diet. Everything we used to think is suddenly wrong.

It never ends.

I firmly believe that food is good. Eating is fun. It's one of the great pleasures of life and contributes to our wellbeing. But you wouldn't think that if you read the alarming diet books and magazine articles and watch the news stories on TV.

By now, everyone has heard and read a million answers to the question "What should I eat?"

That's a great question for selling books and magazines, but it's a horrible question for our happiness, health and vitality. We already know what we should eat. What we want to know is:

1. Why do I eat what I do?

2. How can I want to eat what I should eat?

I'm convinced there is a way to simplify the way we think about health and nutrition. The answers are in our hands.

It's In Our Hands

THE SLOGAN "It's in our hands" has been used in a variety of contexts, but here I use it to mean two main concepts:

First, that we make our own choices—it's up to us; and

Second, that the five hungers, represented by our five fingers, explain both the nutritional challenges we face and the solutions to them.

You use five fingers every time you eat or drink. Once you read this book, you will consider your food choices in a new way. Every time you reach for a beverage, a package, or a fork, you can glance at your hand and ask yourself, which hunger am I satisfying?

Each finger represents one of the five hungers. I've arranged the hungers in order of dominance, starting with the thumb.

Thumb

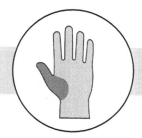

The first digit on our hands is the thumb. The word "thumb" means "swelling" and derives from the same word as tumor and thigh. The opposable nature of the thumb is unique; it's what enables us to write and use tools. This made me think of the unique human ability to design foods that are so appealing as to become irresistible. In a world of abundance, we often eat for pleasure more than need. Therefore, the thumb represents **the first hunger: the hunger for sugar.** The hunger to normalize our body's blood sugar levels is compelling. When we ask ourselves which hunger is driving our desire to eat, we should ask about this hunger first.

Index Finger

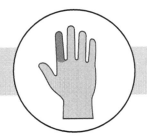

Our second digit, the index finger, is literally our "pointing finger." The word "index" has the same origin as "indicate." And how do we indicate that we're hungry? From an early age, we point to our stomach, indicating with our index finger. Therefore, the index finger represents **the second hunger: the empty stomach, or physical hunger.**

Middle Finger

Our third finger is also our longest. It's in the middle, or center, of the other fingers, just as the third hunger is at the center of our beings. The middle finger reminds me that we can be hungry but not because something tastes good or because our stomachs are empty. Therefore, the middle finger represents **the third hunger: the empty soul, or emotional hunger.**

Ring Finger

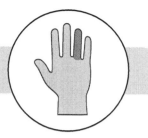

Our fourth digit, the ring finger, gets its name from the tradition of carrying a ring, especially a wedding ring. The Romans wore the wedding ring on the left ring finger on the theory it was closest to the heart and so represented love. In other cultures, the ring finger is the fourth digit on the right hand. Other tokens, such as academic or sports rings, are also commonly worn on the ring finger. The ring finger represents commitment, habits, and goals. Therefore it represents **the fourth hunger: the hunger for stability.**

Pinky

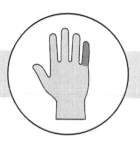

Our final digit, the "pinky," is the smallest of our fingers. It's sort of an outlier; if you put the four fingers together, it's the odd-man-out in an otherwise clear hierarchy. Even in the children's game "little piggy," the pinky toe is the one that runs around screaming. I like to think of the pinky as the fun finger, the one that does its own thing. Therefore, the pinky represents **the fifth hunger: the hunger for novelty.**

Whole Hand

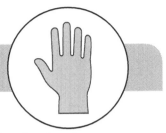

Together, just like the digits on our hands, the five hungers are complementary. They explain most of our actions in life. I'm focusing on food and nutrition in this book, but the five hungers have a broader application.

And I want to emphasize that there's nothing inherently wrong with any of the five hungers. In fact, one of the joys of life is satisfying these hungers, as long as we do so in a positive, productive way. As we'll see, too often when we think we're satisfying a hunger, we're really only making it worse.

The key is identifying each hunger and then remembering them. You don't need to carry around a notebook or consult an app on your phone to remember the five hungers since each one corresponds to one of your fingers. What could be simpler?

While in Cape Town, South Africa, I visited Robben Island. Nelson Mandela had been imprisoned there for eighteen years in a cell smaller than the bathroom in my condo. I reflected on the metaphor that prison represented. How many of my clients, friends, and students have been imprisoned in their own minds and bodies? How many longed for the freedom of health and vitality? Many of them, I knew, had been imprisoned for even longer than eighteen years.

Mandela was prisoner 46664 (prisoner number 466, arriving in 1964). Now there's a clothing line called 46664 that uses the slogan, "It's in our hands" with a logo in the shape of an open hand. When Mandela was finally released from prison and became the President of South Africa, he encouraged everyone, not only in his own country but throughout the world, to recognize that they had the power to make the changes they desired.

And so do you.

What We Want

ONE OF MY HOBBIES when traveling in foreign countries is visiting McDonald's restaurants. This is partly because they usually have free high-speed Internet, but also because it gives me a chance to compare eating habits in the closest thing to a uniform setting.

McDonald's is probably the most sophisticated food seller in history. The story of the company is well known (as are its enormous sales—every day they serve 64 million people). Everywhere I go, the restaurants are busy. Usually they're full of young people, reflecting the potential for a tremendous generational shift in eating habits. Will the rest of the world continue to follow the obesity and health trends we've seen in the United States? I think it's likely. I'll address that in later chapters, but I recognize how easy it is to be a critic, and I'm not going to rehash all the popular criticisms of fast food. For now, I want to look at the implications of us eating what we want.

The McDonald's menu is not uniform around the world. In Buenos Aires, Argentina, for example, I visited a shopping mall with one of the largest food courts I've ever seen. It was so big there were two McDonald's, one at each end in opposite corners (about as far away from each other as possible). Curious at the idea of competing restaurants from the same franchise, we visited both. It turned out that one was kosher. In this context, kosher meant no mixing of dairy and meat. You can't order a cheeseburger at a kosher McDonald's, nor can you get ice cream or a milkshake. They were serious enough about this in Buenos Aires to completely separate the two restaurants.

In Israel, they take a different approach. There, McDonald's has two restaurants within the restaurant, separated by a door, with two sets of cash registers and staff. You still can't get a cheeseburger, but you can order a hamburger from one side, pay, and pick it up, and then go to the other side and order a milkshake or ice cream.

(I visited the world's lowest McDonald's at a resort on the Dead Sea. I have yet to visit the world's highest McDonald's, reportedly located at Cuzco, Peru, at over 11,000 feet.)

The kosher adaptation is far from the only bow to local preferences. My husband visited a McDonald's in Beijing where customers used straws as chop sticks to eat their fries. In Singapore, the fries came with "seaweed seasoning" that looked like finely chopped oregano. In Cape Town, South Africa, I bought a "grilled Chicken Foldover" that used a large wheat flatbread like a tortilla, folded over like a big taco. In France, I bought whole wheat buns for a Big Mac. And, of course, in Hawaii a popular menu item is Spam & Eggs.

I attended a luncheon once at which the speaker was Dean Ornish. Dr. Ornish is president and founder of the nonprofit Preventive Medicine Research Institute in California and the author of several wonderful books on health and nutrition. His most famous is probably *Eat More, Weigh Less*. At our luncheon he described meeting Jack Greenberg, CEO of McDonald's at a conference in Davos, Switzerland. The hosts had seated the two men next to each other, presumably expecting some entertaining conversation. Greenberg asked Ornish why he hated McDonald's so much. Ornish asked Greenberg why McDonald's sold the food they did. The conversation ended up with Greenberg hiring Dr. Ornish to consult on developing healthier foods. Now you can go to McDonald's and buy apple slices in addition to fried potatoes, and McDonald's is by far the largest buyer of apples in the world.

Dr. Ornish eventually consulted with many of the largest food companies and has chaired the health and wellness advisory board of PepsiCo. As he puts it,

> "Although I was initially skeptical, I began to realize that if these companies could use their food technology, celebrities, and resources to make it fun, sexy, hip, crunchy, and convenient to eat more healthfully, this could make a significant difference in the lives of millions of people each day by making it easier for them to eat healthier food, not only in this country but also worldwide . . . . It's easy to be a critic, but I think it's ultimately more productive to help these companies to make healthier foods, which is really to everyone's advantage. It's a little like turning a battleship—it takes a while, but it can go anywhere once it happens." [3]

If the answer is in our hands, and I believe it is, it's critical for us to decide what the question is. In science, we know that the answers we get depend on the questions we ask. It's true in our individual lives as well.

Ultimately, our lives are the answers to one question: what do we really want?

---

3. http://www.huffingtonpost.com/dr-dean-ornish/globalization-of-illnessg_b_558.html

✣ 4 ✣

Full But Hungry

When I was an idealistic college student in the 1970s, my goal was to end world hunger. Starvation was the primary nutrition-related problem. I had heard my whole life about the children starving in India and China. I'd see photos of poverty and hunger that were painful to look at.

Now, forty years later, things have changed. I visit the grocery store and find that many foods have been imported from China. India is a major food exporter. And yet, my goal is still to end world hunger . . . just not in the way I had expected.

You see, around the world, starvation is no longer the primary food-related health problem.

Obesity is.

And obesity is really another form of malnutrition.

It's a failure to address the five hungers.

While I was in college, my youthful idealism took me to rural Colombia for eighteen months on a humanitarian assignment. I was determined to teach the people better health practices, sharing the knowledge and experience I had as an *American Nutrition Expert*. Although we had many successes, we also learned that we didn't know it all. No matter how "advanced" our ways were, there was no way people were going to change their habits on our say-so.

The Colombian people taught me a lesson that I see repeated on a daily basis in the supermarkets, the television shows, the bookstores, and the shopping malls throughout the world. Billions of words, untold hours of speech, and infinite numbers of electrons (not to mention trillions of dollars) have been spent on advice about diet, food, and exercise. No matter how insightful the message, no matter how clever the presentation, no matter how motivating the promised benefits, people still overeat. Americans are no more willing than the rural Colombians to change their habits on someone else's say-so.

And yet, I still think it's possible to end world hunger—which means ending both literal starvation in poor countries and obesity everywhere else.

This book explains how.

Even in today's well-fed world, we are still hungry. We overeat because we are still hungry, even when we're full of food. We just don't recognize the many reasons we eat. I call these the five hungers, but in many ways they are *stealth appetites*. They sneak up on us without revealing their existence until it's too late. We're not defenseless, however. Our most important weapon is our memory, and that's why I use the hand as a reminder.

This book is the opposite of a typical diet book that encourages you to deprive yourself of "bad" food, or follow the latest fad, or lose it all in one week. My focus is on health and happiness, not arbitrary BMI or weight standards. Studies have shown that you can be *thin* and unhealthy. And you can weigh *more* than the charts specify and yet be healthy. People who are slightly overweight actually have lower mortality rates.[4] But if your goal is to lose weight, or

---

4. Janssen, I., (2007) "Morbidity and mortality risk associated with an overweight BMI in older men and women, *Obesity* (Silver Spring), 2007 Jul;15(7):1827-40;
Zajacova, J. & Burgard, S. (2011) "Overweight Adults May Have the Lowest Mortality— Do They Have the Best Health?" *American Journal of Epidemiology*

maintain a desired weight, you don't have to be hungry all the time to accomplish your goal.

Food is not the enemy.

Miseating is.

Notice I wrote "miseating" instead of "overeating." Miseating is not only a valid word in Scrabble and Words with Friends, but a word with which we should all be more familiar. It means eating improperly. I use it to mean eating for the wrong reasons.

When we *miseat*, we will end up "full but hungry."

When we find the real way to satisfy the five hungers, we will stop *miseating*. Our food will be a satisfying reward because it is used for its real purpose, its optimal utility: satisfying true hunger.

Then we'll be full and satisfied.

And I'm pretty sure that's something we all want.

Your Personal Nutrition Calculator

ONCE YOU UNDERSTAND the five hungers, you will have a new way to remember hunger cues. By using your fingers, you have a built-in nutrition calculator with you at all times—the world's first non-electronic app! Whenever you feel like eating, use your fingers to determine what is prompting that feeling. Then you can address it effectively without miseating.

Start with the thumb and think of the need for a normal blood sugar level. Part 1 of this book explains how irregular meal spacing or unbalanced carb intake can lead to fatigue and unpleasant cravings. Assess your meals and decide if it is time for a balanced meal or snack.

Second is the index finger, where you check satiety level and physical emptiness, as explained in Part 2. Rate your hunger on the satiety scale and decide if you need to eat to avoid counterproductive deprivation feelings. Choose foods with low energy density and high nutrient density.

Third, the emotional middle finger can help you assess if your hunger is coming from emotional needs as explained in Part 3. Turn to healthier versions of comfort foods and find alternative ways to feed the emotional emptiness.

Fourth is the ring finger, which can help you assess if your hunger is coming from your habits as explained in Part 4. When you understand how your habits may be fooling you into thinking you need unhealthy foods, you can work on making new habits that work in your favor.

Fifth is the pinky, to help you consider your need for novelty and fun, especially physical movement your body may be craving, as explained in Part 5.

The Five Hunger Check is the new "handmaid of genius" to understand our own hunger.

After you read and understand all five hungers, see Chapter 60 for an example of how the Five Hunger Check can work in a busy person's life.

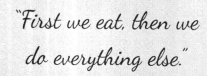

"*First we eat, then we
do everything else.*"

— M. F. K. FISHER —

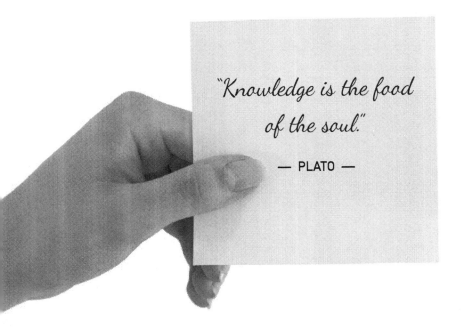

"Knowledge is the food
of the soul."

— PLATO —

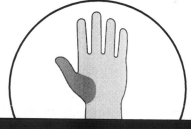

~+~ PART I ~+~

The Thumb

The First Hunger Is for Sugar

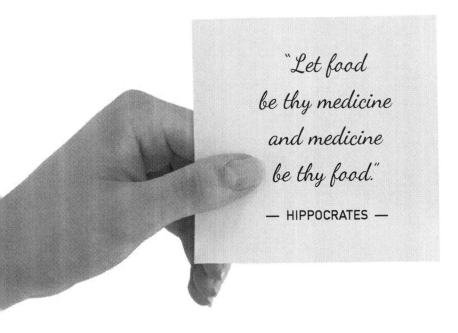

"Let food
be thy medicine
and medicine
be thy food."

— HIPPOCRATES —

✦ 6 ✦

"It's Irresistible"

As a hospital dietitian and community health educator, I have spoken to and counseled thousands of men and women over the years. While everyone is different, I've noticed common patterns in our approaches to food and lifestyle that are reflected in national statistics on food consumption.

We find processed foods—especially sugar—irresistible.

In that sense, we're not much different from other species. Some years ago I was in Malaysia. We visited a park and were soon surrounded by long-armed monkeys begging for food. I noticed they had raided a nearby trash can, cleaning out the remnants of human snacks and candy. One was finishing up a bag of potato chips.

There was abundant food in the trees where they lived. None of these monkeys was exactly starving. But like most of us, they sought the delightful experience of tasting something specifically engineered and processed to appeal to our taste buds. Like ants attracted to picnics, these monkeys had learned that humans brought with them delicacies they'd never find in the jungle.

It's no secret that we like sugar. The average American drinks fifty gallons of sugar-added beverages a year. As a nation, we spend about $56 billion annually on sugary soft drinks.

But it's not sugar, *per se*, that we demand. It's processed sugar. Fresh fruit contains abundant natural sugar, but it comes with many more interesting add-ons, including fiber, vitamins, minerals, phytochemicals, and enzymes.

Not to mention, fruit spoils if you don't eat it.

While there are few if any American households that fall short on sugar consumption, only 23% of households eat the recommended number of fruit servings per day. According to the USDA, low-income households consume even less; food stamp "recipient households tend to consume more meats, added sugars, and total fats."[5]

Many diet and health books focus on the big three diet issues: sugar, fat, and salt. All three contribute important attributes of processed foods, but by far the biggest problem is sugar. Sugar consumption truly stands out like a sore thumb!

---

5. http://www.ers.usda.gov/publications/aer833/aer833.pdf

✦ 7 ✦

The Sweet Sally Syndrome

ONE OF THE MOST common nutrition-related complaints I've heard has been a lack of energy. "I get tired," many women tell me, "and I need something to get me going. Then work is stressful and in the afternoon, and I need another boost."

I know many women who suffer from what I call "The Sweet Sally Syndrome." Sally is my friend who is one of the sweetest people you've ever known—and you also know her well. She's a composite of hundreds of women I've known. In a typical day, she follows this routine:

Sally doesn't sleep well. She wakes up late. She doesn't have time for breakfast, but that's okay because she's not hungry anyway. She grabs her coffee to help her wake up and she's off to work.

By noon, she's starving. She feels justified in having a large lunch of a chicken sandwich and fries, maybe a shake because she skipped breakfast. Maybe even a pie because she worked hard all morning. At least she didn't have a hamburger; that would be fattening!

By mid-afternoon, she's getting sleepy. She drinks a diet cola or two to keep her going.

On the way home she thinks about dinner with a hint of dread. She's too tired to cook, and her family doesn't like waiting anyway, so she stops to pick up pizza on the way home. Later that evening, she craves something sweet. She hasn't eaten that much during the day, really. She only had one slice of pizza. So she deserves a couple of cookies and a dish of ice cream before bed.

She goes to bed but doesn't sleep well again. She knows she has to change something but doesn't know what, exactly, to do.

Finally she makes an appointment with a dietitian (me).

As I listen to her story, I realize she's well-intentioned. She cares about her family, her job, and her health. But the pressures of everyday living have blinded her to the basic biology that explains what she's going through. She's *miseating* and doesn't realize why.

"Let's start with blood sugar," I explain.

What Is Normal Blood Sugar?

Your body consumes blood sugar the way your car consumes gasoline; in fact the fuels are similar—your body burns *carbohydrates* while your car burns *hydrocarbons*. Your body engine, however, never shuts off. Even when you're sitting quietly, just reading or thinking, your body is burning that sugar. Your brain alone burns about 25% of your blood sugar, except when you're exercising.[6] Just as your car warns you when your tank is down to an eighth, your body has a warning system that flashes when your blood sugar gets too low.

The Sweet Sally Syndrome is an excessive rise and fall of blood sugar levels. Sally skipped breakfast, ignoring the warning light. So then at lunch, she filled the tank—and then some. It's as though she held the gas pump and didn't let it click off, spilling gas all over the ground. Except when Sally overeats, the excess gets stored as fat.

Sally's lunch caused another problem. Reacting to the too-low blood sugar, high carbs at lunch caused her blood sugar to jump way too high, so much so that her body secreted extra insulin to process it. What goes up must come down, and the higher the climb, the steeper the fall. She crashed in the afternoon, leaving her feeling sleepy. The pizza helped, but by bedtime, she was in a valley again. The ice cream and cookie merely led to another jump and fall, so she couldn't sleep well. And so it continues.

---

6. http://www.ncbi.nlm.nih.gov/books/NBK22436/

"Here's how the biology works," I say, pulling out my handy chart. "Your body is designed for regular meals, roughly three times a day. Your blood sugar rises and falls within a normal range, like this."

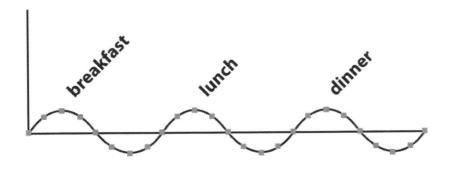

"Except I skip breakfast because I'm losing weight."

I have to admit I used to think the same thing, so I nod. "It's true that consuming fewer calories than you burn will reduce your weight, but you're not doing that, Sally. You're just shifting calories and overcompensating with more later."

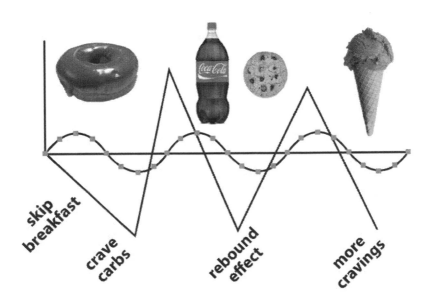

"That high-carb lunch sent your blood sugar on a rocket, but it's going to come back and crash. There's no parachute that's going to save you. And once you crash, you're starving again.

"Plus, look at the extra food you're eating for lunch. You're eating enough for breakfast and lunch combined. You're letting the gas spill over, see?"

"So, I need to stop eating carbs?"

By now I am proud of my self-control, from years of practice refraining from rolling my eyes or smacking my forehead when clients say things like this.

"Not exactly, Sally. I know you probably have a dozen diet books at home that tell you to stay away from carbs. Throw them out. They're wrong. Your body *needs* carbs. Just the right ones, at the right time, in the right amounts.

"And you need to understand carbohydrates."

Understanding Carbohydrates

CARBOHYDRATES ARE poorly understood and accused of being Enemy #1. Many fad diets have claimed that cutting carbs out of your diet can help you create a slender and healthy body because carbs are *bad*. A book published recently was titled *Bread Is the Devil*[7] and reflects the perception that certain foods are the culprits for obesity and need to be avoided at all costs. *Miseating* is the real culprit. In a healthy and balanced diet, carbohydrates can be your friend.

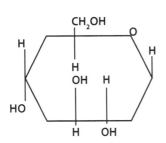

Carbohydrates are all made of carbon, hydrogen, and oxygen that form a ring. The simplest carbs have either just one or two rings, and they are called *sugars*. The simplest sugar of all is the single ring of glucose—the form the bloodstream absorbs and takes to our muscles where it is burned for energy. Other carbs have to be broken down to the glucose ring before being used in the blood.

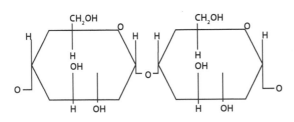

---

7. Bauer, H. & Matthews, K. (2012) Bread Is the Devil: Win the weight loss battle by taking control of your diet demons, St. Martin's Press, New York

A *starch* molecule has the same rings but many more, from 30 to 300 of them attached together. The most complex carbohydrate of all is *fiber*, the same basic structure but with thousands of glucose rings in the same molecule.

Think of carbohydrates as many different foods on a continuum from simple to complex. The whole continuum can be represented by different forms of an apple.

CARBOHYDRATES
Sugar   Starch   Fiber

Simple ⬅--------------➡ Complex

At the simple end is apple juice with complex carbs filtered out. Apple juice is rich in simple sugars; that's why it's always added to juice "blends" so the label can say "100% juice," even though if you look closely, the sugar content is as high as the "fruit punch" drinks made with high fructose corn syrup.

In the middle is applesauce, which essentially consists of mashed apples. Here you have starches along with the natural sugar, but it's not quite as sweet as the apple juice because the proportion of sugar is less than in juice. You have more fiber but less sugar and fewer calories in the same size serving.

Then at the most complex end is the apple itself in its original, natural form. What does nature provide? Sugar, of course; that's what makes fruit attractive to people and animals. You have the same starch as in apple sauce but also more complex carbs (fiber) that your body needs, from the skin.

The apple juice, while delicious, is not going to fill us up for long. The applesauce will last a little longer before we are hungry again. However, the ideal is the original apple, which, because it will take longer to digest, will sustain us for a longer period of time.

If you're working on stabilizing your blood sugar, you need to consider how differently the body treats these three forms of carbohydrates. Sugar is digested immediately and can go straight into the blood stream with its simple six-carbon ring. This rapid absorption makes you hungry again quickly.

If you eat starch (30 to 300 rings), it also has to be broken down into the individual glucose units before being used, so it is absorbed more slowly and stays with you longer. Fiber (800 to 10,000 rings) isn't just slow to digest; it doesn't digest at all—unless you're a cow with four stomachs. The more fiber a food has, the slower the food digests, and the longer it is before you are hungry again.

In addition to the carbs digesting and absorbing, your meals contain protein and fat, which are also slower-digesting and longer-lasting, and tend to moderate blood sugar spikes.

Ideally, each day we would eat three meals at regular intervals with a combination of simple and complex carbs, proteins, and fats, all in moderation.

But you already know that.

As I said from the outset, we know what we should eat. Here's a perfect example. You may have heard of the "5 A Day" program, which the National Cancer Institute started in 1991. The CDC adopted the program in 2005. The idea was to encourage everyone to eat a variety of fruits and vegetables each day. You could drink a cup of apple juice and count it as two servings. But as we've just seen, apple juice is mostly sugar; it's not the equivalent of eating an apple.

In 2007, the CDC changed the program to one called "Fruits & Veggies More Matters."[8] While technically more accurate, it's also more complex. When is the last time you went to the CDC Web site and filled in the box with your age, gender, and amount of physical activity to determine how many fruits and vegetables you need?

That's what I thought.

Your diet isn't an exercise in nuclear physics. To avoid *miseating*, you just need to remember the five hungers and how to properly satisfy each of them.

Let's look at a few common ways in which people try to satisfy the first hunger by *miseating*, getting the wrong kinds of carbs, or eating at the wrong times.

---

8. http://www.fruitsandveggiesmatter.gov/index.html

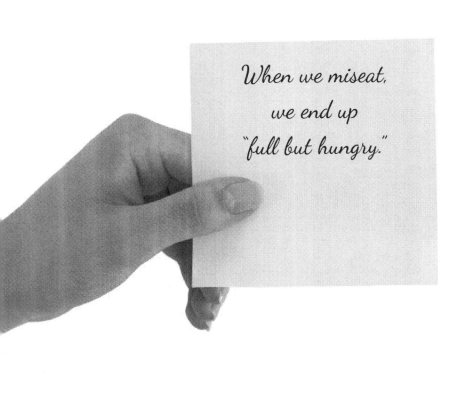

When we miseat,
we end up
"full but hungry."

Blood Sugar Battles

MAINTAINING APPROPRIATE blood sugar levels is a battle, not a skirmish. It's tough work, and we must remain vigilant. The enemy comes in many forms, can strike at any time, and has us surrounded. But we can prevail by learning the enemy's tactics and practicing our defenses.

The Everyday Villain: Soft Drinks

One of the most insidious harms to blood sugar comes in the form of soft drinks. Some children get most of their energy needs from the empty calories of sugary drinks. Even some healthy sounding drinks, such as Sunny Delight, Hawaiian Punch, and Hi-C, are mostly sugar.

I have heard health researchers asserting that "soft drinks are the cigarettes of the obesity epidemic." Barry Popkin, at the University of North Carolina in Chapel Hill suggested that we might consider treating soft drinks like cigarettes by requiring warning labels or taxing them.[9] Carbonated beverages have several similarities to cigarettes: they are marketed heavily to children, are very habit forming, have no redeeming nutritional value, are harmful to your

---

9. Brownell, K., Popkin, B., et al (2009) "The Public Health and Economic Benefits of Taxing Sugar-Sweetened Beverages," *New England Journal of Medicine* 361(16):1599-1605

health, and customers usually become addicted while young and stay loyal all their lives.

According to the Yale Rudd Center, "In 2004, soda companies produced more than 52 gallons of carbonated beverages for each person in the United States, enough for every American to drink one and a half cans every day."[10] Americans now drink twice as much soda as they did in 1972.

The problem has not gone unnoticed. Many school districts ban the sale of soda at schools. Some ban the sale of these drinks only during lunchtime. The Mayor of New York City proposed the ban of sugared soda in containers larger than 16 ounces, based on studies that show people drink all the contents of a container regardless of how large it is.

The debate over the impact of soft drinks is far from over. Coca-Cola's North American Vice President has said "There is no scientific evidence that connects sugary beverages to obesity," while a former marketing executive at Coca-Cola has said, "It took me ten years to figure out that I have a large karmic debt to pay for the number of Cokes I sold across this country." He explained that his marketing objectives focused on how to "drive more ounces into more bodies more often."

Regardless of the ultimate political responses to the competing claims, and without focusing on any one company or product, it's important to make an informed decision for your personal health.

Here are some serious reasons you should consider limiting soft drinks:

- It is easy to consume large amounts of sugar without being conscious of how much you are ingesting.

- The heavy sugar load often causes blood sugar to spike.

---

10. http://www.yaleruddcenter.org/what_we_do.aspx?id=98

- Liquid calories do not provide satiety or fullness (see Part 2).

- Cola drinks contain phosphoric acid for a stronger fizz, which, in turn, is associated with lower bone density and more osteoporosis.[11]

- Many soft drinks contain caffeine, which is habit-forming and has additional side effects when taken in excess (see section on caffeine).

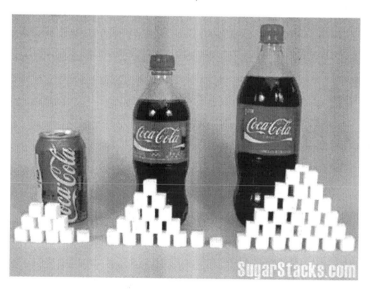

At Sugar Stacks,[12] a Web site that demonstrates how much sugar is in specific foods, you can see in the form of sugar cubes how much sugar you are consuming when you drink a soda or eat a piece of pie. Each cube represents one teaspoon of sugar.

Here's a revealing experiment. Instead of drinking a 20-ounce

---

11. Tucker, K et al, (2006) Colas, but not other carbonated beverages, are associated with low bone mineral density in older women: The Framingham Osteoporosis Study, American Journal of Clinical Nutrition 84(4) 936-942

12. http://www.sugarstacks.com/

bottle of soda next time, try eating 16½ sugar cubes and see how you feel. You probably did not realize you were taking that much sugar in at once.

Even in drinks marketed as healthy, such as SoBe, sugar is the main ingredient. Chocolate milk is high in sugar, contrary to popular misconceptions, Slurpees are not just ice and water, and energy drinks are not low-sugar alternatives to soda pop.

The Villain with Superpowers: Energy Drinks

The surging popularity of energy drinks warrants a separate caution. Four cases of deaths and five cases of seizures were recently documented, all associated with consumption of so-called energy or power drinks.[13] A *New York Times* article cited additional reports of a 28-year-old with a cardiac arrest, an 18-year-old who died playing basketball after drinking Red Bull, and four individuals with bipolar disorder who experienced mania.[14]

After an Australian study, authors warned that even one can of Red Bull could increase heart attack or stroke risk, even in otherwise healthy young people.[15] Notwithstanding that Red Bull is banned in Uruguay, Denmark, and Norway because of health risks, the drinks are enormously popular and sales are over 3.5 billion cans per year in 143 countries.

The Energy Counterfeit: Caffeine

If you are trying to level out your blood sugar you should also review your caffeine use. The *only* source of true energy in the

---

13. Higgins, J., Tuttle, T., Higgins, C., (2010) "Energy Beverages: Content and Safety" *Mayo Clinic Proceedings*, 85(11): 1033-41

14. Brody, J. (2011) "Scientists See Dangers in Energy Drinks" *The New York Times*, 31 January 2011

15. Taylor, R. (2008) "Red Bull drink lifts stroke risk: Australian Study" *Reuters* 14 August 2008

muscles is glucose, but many people tell me they get energy, or at least *feel energized,* with caffeine. They are feeling the stimulant effect of the drug rather than supplying energy to the body.

Although caffeine can be very beneficial if used occasionally, many Americans use it daily and excessively. Such use both removes its benefits and greatly increases its side effects.

Caffeine is the most widely-used psychoactive drug in the world. It can work as a wonder drug, reducing the sensation of fatigue, relieving pain, and increasing alertness. The drawback is that tolerance and adaptation develop quickly, meaning that its effects fade with overuse and the body comes to expect and crave it.[16]

How much is overuse? Since caffeine is so popular and so widely-used, a safe and moderate intake has been widely debated. The U.S. Food and Drug Administration and the American Medical Association consider that a moderate intake at a level that is "generally recognized as safe" equals 200 to 300 mg per day.[17]

It is difficult to specify a "safe" level because people react differently to caffeine. In addition, caffeine content in soft drinks, coffee, and tea varies. As a general guideline, the upper limit of the safe range is equal to about two cups of coffee per day.[18] However, some people can show signs of addiction to caffeine with as little as one cup of coffee a day.[19]

Below are some comparisons with other common beverages to the upper limit of the safe range for caffeine intake. The following contain caffeine approximately equal to two cups of coffee:

---

16. Winston, P. et al (2005) Neuropsychiatric effects of caffeine. *Advances in Psychiatric Treatment* 11:432-439

17. Kovacs, B. What are the sources of caffeine, *Caffeine. MedicineNet.com* Available at http://www.medicinenet.com/caffeine/article.htm

18. Ibid

19. Juliano, L.M., and R.R. Griffiths. "A Critical Review of Caffeine Withdrawal: Empirical Validation of Symptoms and Signs, Incidence, Severity, and Associated Features," *Psychopharmacology* (Berl). Sept, 21, 2004

3 cups of tea (40 to 120 mg per cup)

2¼ 20-oz bottles Mountain Dew (90 mg per 20 oz)

3 20-oz bottles Dr Pepper (68 mg per 20 oz)

3 20-oz bottles Sunkist Orange Soda (68 mg per 20 oz)

3 20-oz bottles Pepsi (63 mg per 20 oz)

3½ 20-oz bottles of CocaCola (58 mg per 20 oz)

5 20-oz bottles Snapple Iced Tea (42 mg per 20 oz)

6 20-oz bottles Barq's Root Beer (38 mg per 20 oz) [20]

25 6-oz cups of hot chocolate (8 mg per 6 oz)

If you are using caffeine daily and experiencing any of the common symptoms of caffeine excess such as anxiety, insomnia, higher blood pressure, increased hot flashes in menopause, to name a few, you should consider replacing your caffeine drinks with another beverage.

The Camouflaged Nemesis: White Flour

Historically, wheat was essential to civilization because of its productivity and long storage life. It's no less important today; worldwide, it's the most heavily traded crop. It's also nutritious, with protein, fat, carbs, minerals, and vitamins. The problem: we often remove the good stuff.

Have you ever had pancakes or cereal for breakfast, a sandwich for lunch, cookies for snacks, spaghetti for dinner, and maybe a piece of cake for dessert?

You're most likely eating refined wheat flour all day long.

In 2010, despite trends toward healthier foods, Americans still bought more loaves of white bread than wheat. (Total dollar sales of whole wheat bread exceeded sales of white bread because wheat bread costs more.)

---

20. Varies with bottling location, sometimes does not contain caffeine; check label

This statistic reflects a general trend toward products that are marketed as "natural" or "whole grain." The message is sinking in: we need whole grains.

Right?

Not so fast.

Let me emphasize right up front: there's nothing wrong with bread, white or otherwise. As I've said, carbs are not "bad" or something you should avoid. It's a question of whether we are *miseating* them.

Bread has long been a staple human food. In revolutionary France, peasants would spend as much as half of their income for bread. Bread is so fundamental that many countries even today subsidize it. In Egypt, over 75% of the people rely on subsidized bread, which costs less than a penny a loaf. Fear of rising bread prices contributed to the collapse of the Mubarak regime.

In most developed countries, we're not at risk of running out of bread, but we have another "bread problem."

When confronted with mobs of French citizens who were starving because they had no bread, Marie Antoinette famously replied, "Let them eat cake!" In her palace, she had no shortage of cake; she couldn't imagine that the peasants had none. The historical accuracy of the statement is questionable—it originated in Jean-Jacques Rousseau's autobiography, which is full of invention—but the concept resonates because it reflects an almost universal human trait.

When we're rich, we eat "better."

Whether the Queen of France uttered the famous phrase or not, kings and queens have always preferred refined wheat products (white bread and cake) over coarse "country" bread. Refined wheat products are easier to chew and digest. They are "sweeter" than whole grain products. To this day, in France you can visit a "Boulangerie" or bread store, or else you can visit a "Patisserie" or pastry store. They call whole wheat bread "pain du compagne" or "country bread."

McDonald's in France offers a Big Mac on whole wheat buns which they call "pain complet" or "complete bread."

"Complete bread" is a wonderful way to express the truth that whole grains are "complete" while refined grains are not.

Fortunately, we have many options now. We can buy whole grain spaghetti, pancake mixes, breads, and other grain-based products.

Unfortunately, too often we go for the white stuff.

Remember our discussion of carbohydrate chains? The refining process cuts those chains into smaller portions. It shifts the flour closer to the sugar end of the spectrum.

Refined white bread is to whole wheat bread what apple juice is to apples.

Just as it is okay to drink apple juice from time to time, eating refined flour occasionally isn't going to hurt you. But there's a reason we have birthday cake only once a year.

I once heard Dr. John McDougall speak, advocating a very strict vegetarian diet with few sugars and fats.[21] One woman in the audience said, "That would be no fun at all. Don't you ever get to celebrate, even on your birthday?" Dr. McDougall replied, "Oh yes, I enjoy a wonderful birthday cake and think everyone should. The problem is that Americans eat as if every day is their birthday!"

Remember that white flour digests like a simple carbohydrate, breaking down quickly to send glucose to the bloodstream. Add to that a nice frosting (donuts, cupcakes, birthday cakes), or syrup (pancakes and waffles), or jelly or jam (toast, sandwiches, Danish) and you've got an explosion of sugar.

Kids today might not believe there was a time when PopTarts came without frosting, but when I was young, the filling alone was more than enough sugar!

In fact, in many cases white flour is nothing more than a delivery system for even more pure sugar.

Which leads me to the next topic.

21. See http://www.drmcdougall.com

Delivery Systems

If the first hunger was solely for sugar, we could satisfy it with spoonfuls of pure sugar. Maybe when you were young, you opened those packets at the restaurant and poured the whole thing in your mouth. It was a fun experiment but you didn't repeat it often, if ever.

Why?

Because isolated, sugar is not palatable.

Sugar forms tiny granules. It's like eating sand. It's not a pleasant texture and the grains stick in our teeth. We like the sugary taste, but we prefer other textures, so the food industry has developed a variety of delivery systems. Check that. The "food industry" is too generic a name. Actually, there are thousands of food scientists hard at work, developing ingenious delivery systems designed to penetrate all your defenses. It's a complex field. Here's how one university describes its program:

> Nutritional science draws upon the chemical, biological, and social sciences to understand the complex relationships between human health, nutritional status, food, and lifestyle patterns, and social and institutional environments. Understanding these relationships includes the study of the metabolic regulation, biochemistry, and function of nutrients, nutrient requirements throughout the life span, the role of diet in reducing risk of chronic disease, the nutritional quality of foods, and interventions and policies designed to promote the nutritional health of individuals, communities, and populations.[22]

That describes the aspirations of the good guys in this battle, but it also gives some insight into the level of sophistication involved in food design.

---

22. http://courses.cornell.edu/content.php?catoid=12&navoid=2188

Look at one of the most popular sugar delivery systems in history: the Oreo cookie. Kraft (owner of Nabisco) reports that 70 million Oreos are consumed every day around the world. That's enough for about four Oreos for every single human on the planet (at a population of 8 billion) every year.

Oreos were first released in 1912 in Manhattan. Now the Oreo cookie has over 26 million Facebook fans.

The company promoted their 100th birthday with a Web page that suggested a novel reason for eating the cookie: "In a world that's become far too adult, a couple of Oreo cookies, a glass of milk, and a shared Twist, Lick and Dunk is all it takes to set your inner kid loose. Celebrate the kid inside all of us."[23]

You can get the original Oreo or several variations. For example, "OREO Fudge Cremes are a thin, crispy OREO cookie topped with unmistakable OREO creme, wrapped in fudge." They come in Original, Mint, Peanut Butter crème, and Golden Oreo in the United States.

A single serving of Double Stuf Oreos (29 grams) contains 140 calories and 13 grams of sugar; 13 grams of sugar have only 50 calories, so where does the rest come from? 60 calories are from fat.

In other words, these cookies deliver more fat calories than sugar calories.

You can buy reduced fat Oreos instead. A serving of these (34 grams) contains only 40 calories from fat, but they contain a little more sugar—14 grams.

As a sugar delivery system, the Oreo is effective. The number one ingredient is sugar. Number two is refined wheat flour, followed by oil and high fructose corn syrup.

A gram of sugar contains about 4 calories, so you're actually consuming more calories by eating an Oreo than you would if you

---

23. http://www.nabiscoworld.com/oreo/

ate the same amount of pure sugar, thanks to the fats in the delivery system.

Oreos are popular because the delivery system provides so many sensations. The crust is crispy. The filling is creamy. There are no unpleasant granules. We can dip them in milk and enjoy a different texture. We can crumble them onto ice cream. Oreos are one of the most perfect—and perfected—sugar delivery systems known to mankind.

Quite an accomplishment.

But there are many other delivery systems.

We've looked at a few of these already. Soft drinks deliver sugar through a pleasant liquid, preferably cold, with a little fizz in it. Energy drinks, coffee, and tea add massive doses of caffeine along with different flavors. Flour in all its forms, combined with fats and salts, can deliver sugar in infinite varieties.

Pet food scientists describe palatability as a function of how much an animal is attracted to the flavor, aroma, and texture of a food. These are the same factors used to design sugar delivery systems.

As sophisticated as the food companies are, we're not defenseless.

We have a thumb.

Take a minute, right now, and look at your thumb.

Wiggle it a little. Bend it. It's nodding, agreeing that the next time you pick up a sugar delivery system, it will remind you to ask yourself if you're responding to the first hunger—the hunger for sugar.

If so, how are you going to respond?

11

How to Stabilize Blood Sugar

SALLY IS LIKE many people I know whose dramatic swings and frequent fatigue and cravings suggest blood sugar out of control.

There are several ways to help the blood sugar stay at an optimal stable level. It is important to remember that these are not hard and fast rules, but variable and individual. You need to find out what works best for you. Get to know what is normal for your blood sugar levels. Once you do, you (and your health care provider if necessary) can create an individualized plan to help you keep your blood sugar level under control.

Sally's first mistake in her blood sugar battle was trying to skip a meal or deprive herself, with the thought that she needed to lose weight by cutting back. She has the idea that starving herself will be heroic, will prove she has will-power, will save calories and will help her lose weight. She is sadly mistaken! The deprivation feelings set off a protective survival mechanism, while the low blood sugar causes carbohydrate cravings. Instead of helping her lose weight, the deprivation feelings are more likely to reinforce the vicious cycle of overeating and starving.

Breakfast

The first, most basic thing you can do to prevent these swings is to eat a healthy breakfast. Without breakfast, you may have not just a moderate valley, but a dramatic drop, leading to cravings for sugar. Blood sugar levels are usually lowest in the morning, before the first meal of the day, and rise after meals for an hour or two. If you miss breakfast, you are more likely, as with Sally in our case study, to grab high sugar foods to satisfy your hunger. Your blood sugar will peak quickly, but then drop just as quickly, leaving you hungry once more. This vicious cycle can be repeated all day long.

Not hungry in the morning? You do not have to eat the minute you roll out of bed, but try to have at least something in the first two hours after getting up. It can be small, like a piece of fruit and as your body gets used to eating in the morning, work up to a larger breakfast.

In a rush, no time to eat? Keep on hand some fast-grab breakfast foods that are easy to eat even as you run out the door or on your drive to work: an apple or banana, string cheese, drinkable yogurt.

Ready for a bigger breakfast? If you plan ahead, you have time to make a healthy meal that will help you all day. Try to include at a minimum both complex carbs and protein such as:

- Yogurt and fruit, whole grain muffin
- Whole grain cereal and milk
- Scrambled egg and wheat toast
- Cottage cheese and fruit
- Peanut butter on whole wheat toast

No Deprivation

If you are trying to control blood sugar, deprivation is your worst enemy. Not only does deprivation set off the protective survival mechanism, it causes carbohydrate cravings and leads to self-defeating starve/binge cycles. Plan ahead with healthy snacks you may need—remember, the goal is to avoid feeling deprived!

Evenly Spaced Meals and Snacks

Ideally we would eat regularly spaced meals all day long, eating perfectly planned meals like clockwork. Unfortunately, our lives rarely give us that luxury. But we can work toward the goal of eating at regular times, and plan snacks to help make the schedule work.

What time are you likely to eat breakfast? Plan a lunch four to five hours later, with dinner four to five hours after that. If you know it will be longer than five hours before the next meal, fit a small snack in the middle.

Change Your Food Outlook

Michael Pollan, in his excellent book *The Omnivore's Dilemma*, described a compound paradox:

> We show our surprise at this [people eating "unhealthy" food but being healthy] by speaking of something called the "French paradox," for how could a people who eat such demonstrably toxic substances as foie gras and triple crème cheese actually be slimmer and healthier than we are? Yet I wonder if it doesn't make more sense to speak in terms of an American paradox—that is, a notably unhealthy people obsessed by the idea of eating healthily.[24]

It's not merely a "French paradox," of course. People in many cultures enjoy "rich" foods without gaining weight or deteriorating health. The answers are not found in what is eaten but how it is eaten. The healthy people are the ones who don't miseat.

Curious about the premise that the French are famous for enjoying fattening food, I've traveled to France to observe how people eat and live. My observations verify the statistics: the French people as a whole

24. Pollan, M., (2006) *The Omnivore's Dilemma: A Natural History of Four Meals,* The Penguin Press, New York, page 3

are not fat. *The Omnivore's Dilemma* mentions this in passing, but several books have been written about why this is the case.

French author, Mireille Guiliano, in her #1 bestseller *French Women Don't Get Fat,* explained several key factors in the French women's ability to say slim:

- Smaller portion sizes

- Savoring food to increase the feeling of satisfaction, choosing a small amount of high quality food (like a good chocolate) rather than larger amounts of low quality food

- Eating three meals a day and not snacking

- Taking in plenty of liquid such as water, herbal tea and soup

- Sitting down and eating mindfully, not multitasking and eating while standing up, watching TV, or reading

- Emphasizing freshness, variety, balance, and, above all, pleasure

These are each important factors that I'll discuss later (they each fit within the five hungers), but she didn't point out the most obvious factor.

The French have tamed their hunger for sugar. For example, the French drink far more wine than Americans, and much less soda. One study showed that while the per capita soft drink consumption in the U.S. is 216 liters, in France it's only 37.2 liters.[25] A standard drink of red wine contains 1 gram of sugar, while a standard cola drink contains 33 grams. Even a 750 ml bottle of red wine contains only 5 grams of sugar.

---

25. Euromonitor International, cited in http://www.nationmaster.com/graph/foo_sof_dri_con-food-soft-drink-consumption#source

Rescue Yourself from Soft Drinks

You can get used to other beverages to replace soft drinks, but it may be a difficult transition. Here are some ways to find more energy without caffeine or the sugar rush you might be used to:

- Improve your sleep patterns. Be aware that your sleep may be greatly affecting your energy level, which you may be trying to self-medicate with food instead of working on getting effective sleep. Caffeine use can in turn be making insomnia worse. Many resources are available to improve your sleep, such as those from the *National Sleep Foundation*.[26] In addition to expert references and a guide to resource books on sleep, they publish a list of guidelines that can improve your *sleep hygiene*.[27]

- Increase your level of physical activity. Too many of us lack exercise and make up for it by overeating (see Part 5).

The best beverage to satisfy thirst is water. If you're drinking something else, make sure you recognize that you're feeding one of the hungers, not quenching your thirst.

Consider using 100% fruit juice as a transition to drinking more water. Recognize, however, that fruit juices also contain simple sugars, so it is easy to over-consume without realizing it. Even better is to eat the whole fruit. Consider cutting back on sugar by progressively diluting your fruit juice with water until you are just flavoring your water with a little fruit. Yes, you can get used to it!

Parents especially need to recognize that children often overdo fruit juice. Although 100% fruit juice is healthier than soft drinks,

---

26. See http://www.sleepfoundation.org/
27. Thorpy, M. (2003) "Sleep Hygiene" Ask the Expert, National Sleep Foundation. Available at http://www.sleepfoundation.org/article/ask-the-expert/sleep-hygiene.

the American Academy of Pediatrics suggests ways to limit juice as follows: [28]

- No juice for infants under 6 months of age
- Infants 6 to 12 months: up to 4 to 6 oz juice per day in a cup
- Children age 1 to 6 years: up to 4 to 6 oz juice per day
- Older children: 8 to 12 oz juice per day
- Encourage whole fruits instead of juice

---

28. American Academy of Pediatrics. Policy Statement, The Use and Misuse of Fruit Juice in Pediatrics. Pediatrics Vol. 107 No. 5 May 2001, pp. 1210-1213

✦ 12 ✦

Sweet Sally's Makeover

Let's revisit our case study. We are going to find solutions for Sally so that she will not suffer from the fatigue and cravings she did before. When blood sugar is controlled, it is so much easier to appreciate food as the gift and blessing it is.

Remember to find solutions that work for you. Here are just a few of hundreds of possible options for Sally's Lifestyle Makeover.

Sally sleeps soundly because she took the advice from the National Sleep Foundation[29] and wakes up early to take a walk.

She has time for a quick breakfast before work, consisting of wheat toast with peanut butter and a slice of cantaloupe.

She starts dinner in her Crock-Pot: in just five minutes she throws in ingredients for black bean chili.

She packs her lunch and snacks, so in the mid-morning she has finger food ready: cucumber slices with bean dip.

At lunch she has a chopped salad with tuna, and a pear. Since she brought her lunch and did not have to drive down the street to buy it, she has time for a pleasant walk before returning to her desk.

In the mid-afternoon she has another snack of baby carrots and snow peas.

---

29. Thorpy, M. (2003) "Sleep Hygiene" *Ask the Expert, National Sleep Foundation.* Available at http://www.sleepfoundation.org/article/ask-the-expert/sleep-hygiene

She gets home to dinner all prepared: Crock-Pot chili with peaches for dessert.

That evening she treats herself to a fruit smoothie before bed, adding in some tofu to make it creamy and provide some protein.

No caffeine in her system, Sally sleeps soundly to awake refreshed the next day.

13

Check Your Diabetes Risk

THE INCIDENCE OF Type 2 Diabetes is rapidly increasing in a pattern consistent with the erratic eating that characterizes modern hectic lifestyles.

If you suspect significant blood sugar highs and lows, you can take a simple Diabetes Risk Test to help decide if you need to consult your health care provider.

This test is provided by the American Diabetes Association, which also offers a wealth of background information and resources at www.diabetes.org. There is an online interactive version on their Web site, or you can add up your risk on the chart that follows.

If you score 5 or higher, check with a health care provider to see if additional testing is needed.

If you've been diagnosed with diabetes of any kind be sure to follow your doctor's guidance regarding all aspects of your diet.

ARE YOU AT RISK FOR
TYPE 2 **DIABETES?**

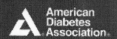
American Diabetes Association.

Diabetes Risk Test

1 How old are you?
  Less than 40 years (0 points)
  40—49 years (1 point)
  50—59 years (2 points)
  60 years or older (3 points)

Write your score in the box.

2 Are you a man or a woman?
  Man (1 point)   Woman (0 points)

3 If you are a woman, have you ever been diagnosed with gestational diabetes?
  Yes (1 point)   No (0 points)

4 Do you have a mother, father, sister, or brother with diabetes?
  Yes (1 point)   No (0 points)

5 Have you ever been diagnosed with high blood pressure?
  Yes (1 point)   No (0 points)

6 Are you physically active?
  Yes (0 points)   No (1 point)

7 What is your weight status?
  (see chart at right)

Add up your score.

Height	Weight (lbs.)		
4' 10"	119-142	143-190	191+
4' 11"	124-147	148-197	198+
5' 0"	128-152	153-203	204+
5' 1"	132-157	158-210	211+
5' 2"	136-163	164-217	218+
5' 3"	141-168	169-224	225+
5' 4"	145-173	174-231	232+
5' 5"	150-179	180-239	240+
5' 6"	155-185	186-248	247+
5' 7"	159-190	191-254	255+
5' 8"	164-196	197-261	262+
5' 9"	169-202	203-269	270+
5' 10"	174-208	209-277	278+
5' 11"	179-214	215-285	286+
6' 0"	184-220	221-293	294+
6' 1"	189-226	227-301	302+
6' 2"	194-232	233-310	311+
6' 3"	200-239	240-318	319+
6' 4"	205-245	246-327	328+
	(1 Point)	(2 Points)	(3 Points)

You weigh less than the amount in the left column (0 points)

If you scored 5 or higher:

You are at increased risk for having type 2 diabetes. However, only your doctor can tell for sure if you do have type 2 diabetes or prediabetes (a condition that precedes type 2 diabetes in which blood glucose levels are higher than normal). Talk to your doctor to see if additional testing is needed.

Type 2 diabetes is more common in African Americans, Hispanics/Latinos, American Indians, and Asian Americans and Pacific Islanders.

For more information, visit us at
www.diabetes.org or call 1-800-DIABETES

Adapted from Bang et al, Ann Intern Med 151:775-783, 2009. Original algorithm was validated without gestational diabetes as part of the model.

Visit us on Facebook
Facebook.com/AmericanDiabetesAssociation

Lower Your Risk

The good news is that you can manage your risk for type 2 diabetes. Small steps make a big difference and can help you live a longer, healthier life.

If you are at high risk, your first step is to see your doctor to see if additional testing is needed.

Visit diabetes.org or call 1-800-DIABETES for information, tips on getting started, and ideas for simple, small steps you can take to help lower your risk.

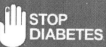
STOP DIABETES

14

FingerTIPS about the First Hunger

"Thumbnail" sketch of managing blood sugar

- A hectic lifestyle may be keeping you from healthy blood sugar levels if you skip breakfast, go for long periods without eating, then eat high-sugar and high-fat meals.

- Low blood sugar often causes fatigue and carbohydrate cravings.

- Carbohydrates are not the enemy and are an important part of a healthy diet.

- The simplest carbs are sugars that digest quickly.

- Starch is made of many simple sugars connected in the same molecule.

- Fiber is the most complex carb, made of thousands of simple sugars. It lasts longer in the digestive tract so your blood sugar does not dip as fast.

- Soft drinks are a common way of taking in too many sugars quickly without getting filled up. Fruit juices are better but still should be limited since they are also high in sugar. Even better is a whole piece of fruit.

- Caffeine is a stimulant that can give the feeling of energy, but tolerance and adaptation develop quickly. It is easy to overuse caffeine.

- White flour is a refined carb that digests quickly and does not keep blood sugar as level as whole grains and other foods high in complex carbs (fiber).

- Evenly-spaced meals will help control blood sugar. Try to go no longer than five hours between meals, or schedule a small snack if the interval will be longer than five hours.

- Foods that will help control blood sugar include more complex carbs and fewer sugars eaten together with proteins and healthy fats.

- Take the Diabetes Risk Test to see if you need to consult your health care provider about your blood sugar control.

⊹ 15 ⊹

Resources about Blood Sugar

HERE ARE SOME helpful books and articles to explore for more information as you become more aware of the first hunger.

American Diabetes Association, *"MyFoodAdvisor: Recipes for Healthy Living,"* available at http://bit.ly/myfoodadvisor

> A free online resource with recipes, cooking tips and a meal plan to follow, appropriate for those managing diabetes and anyone interested in controlling blood sugar. Registering online (free) gives access to daily meal plans, recipes and other tools.

Fries, Wendy C., (2011), *"13 Ways to Fight Sugar Cravings"* WebMD Feature available at http://bit.ly/fightcravings

> Ideas and tips for sensible and healthy ways to deal with cravings.

Fittante, Ann, (2006), *The Sugar Solution: Your Symptoms are Real and Your Solution is Here,* Prevention Magazine

> Tools to identify and correct high blood sugar and drop excess pounds, replenish energy stores and reduce disease risk.

Kessler, David A., (2009) *The End of Overeating: Taking Control of the Insatiable American Appetite,* Rodale, New York

> Describes the way the food industry designs, manufactures, advertises,and distributes foods that stimulate our appetites to the point we lose control over our eating habits.

Pollan, Michael, (2006), *The Omnivore's Dilemma: A Natural History of Four Meals,* Penguin Press, New York

> Provides answers to the question "What should we have for dinner?" by examining in detail where our food comes from, comparing natural to processed foods.

16

FingerFOODS
Recipe for the First Hunger

IN A RUSH to provide balanced meals for yourself or your family, to better control blood sugar levels? You don't have to resort to the drive-thru. In less than five minutes in the morning you can put together this hearty meal that will be ready for you at the end of your busy day.

Crock-Pot Vegetarian Chili in a Flash

2 16-oz cans black beans
1 16-oz can kidney beans
2 14.5-oz cans tomato sauce
2 Tbsp dried minced onions
2 1.25-oz pkgs chili seasoning
   (or your own seasoning mix made in advance)

Stir together all ingredients in Crock-Pot. Cook on low
   setting 8 to 12 hours.
Serve with optional toppings:
- Grated cheese
- Sour cream
- Fritos (corn chips)
Makes 10 1-cup servings.

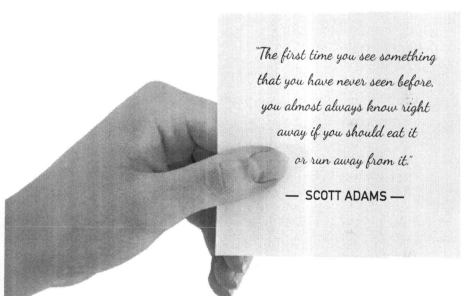

"The first time you see something that you have never seen before, you almost always know right away if you should eat it or run away from it."

— SCOTT ADAMS —

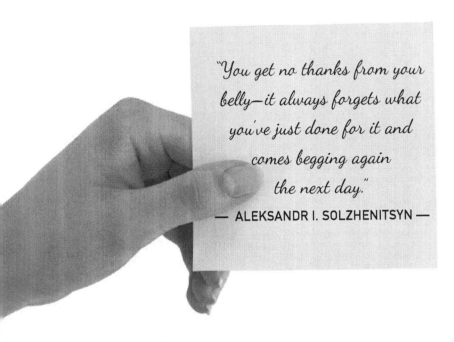

"You get no thanks from your belly—it always forgets what you've just done for it and comes begging again the next day."

— ALEKSANDR I. SOLZHENITSYN —

PART II

The Index Finger

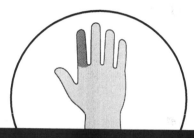

The Second Hunger Is for Physical Emptiness

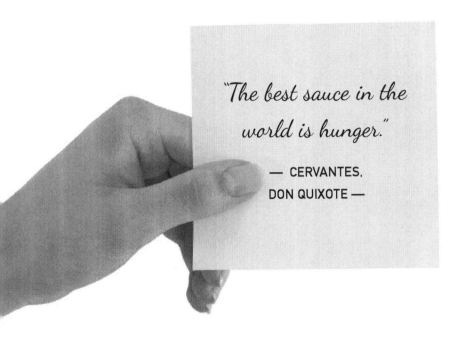

"The best sauce in the world is hunger."

— CERVANTES,
DON QUIXOTE —

17

What a Mother Knows

AS A MOTHER of three teenage boys (my daughter was quite different), I often wondered if they had anything but a stomach inside of them. I would watch them eat in amazement. Theoretically, an average adult stomach has a volume of about 1/3 cup, expandable to 4 cups or more.

Yet it seemed like my boys could consume a couple of gallons worth of food at one sitting.

At least.

They were like human vacuum cleaners.

And no matter how much they ate, they didn't seem to put on any weight. If I had eaten half as much as they did, I would have gained five pounds a month.

Watching them eat was a dramatic contrast to the patients I had in the hospital, most of whom were women fighting with eating disorders. They didn't want to eat, but they felt compelled to do so. I began inquiring into the physics of hunger, a topic we didn't discuss much in school.

I wondered, is there a physical component to hunger? Do our brains register hunger only because our blood sugar is low, or are there triggers based on physical emptiness?

Thinking about my sons and their insatiable hunger, the phrase "nature abhors a vacuum" came to mind. I wondered where the phrase came from. It turns out Aristotle is credited with observing that "nature abhors a vacuum." He was trying to explain motion, proposing that when an object moves, it leaves behind empty space, or a vacuum, which sucks in liquids or air and pushes the object forward.

Aristotle's theory was eventually rejected as a matter of physics, but the principle finds application (at least by analogy) to our stomachs.

It's not just teenage boys who know what an empty stomach feels like. We all "abhor a vacuum" when it occurs inside us!

18

Lessons from the French

IN 2011, my husband and I were on a small island off the coast of Brittany in France, shopping in a grocery store for cheese and crackers. I noticed an unusual candy bar (okay, so I wasn't blind to the goodies) and sneaked it into our cart. Only later, when I went to unwrap it, did I notice the "instructions" on the back. I was supposed to eat one square with a balanced meal.

One square?

There were twelve squares in this (relatively small) chocolate bar and I was supposed to eat one of them? If I did that, my husband

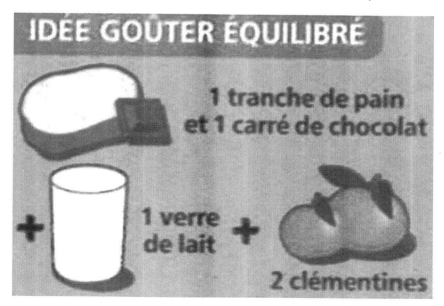

would eat the remaining eleven. How could anyone eat only one square?

The answer was also in the nutrition labeling. It suggested I should eat a couple of clementines, a glass of milk, and a piece of bread along with my one square of chocolate.

Ah-hah!

The nefarious fruit industry had infiltrated the candy industry and sales of clementines were booming!

Unfortunately, we hadn't bought any clementines, so I violated the instructions and ate my single square of chocolate "sans le fruit." But someone (I presume the French government had something to do with the label) had a point. If I had followed their instructions, I couldn't have eaten more than one square of chocolate. Possibly two. But that would have meant eating four clementines, two pieces of bread, and two glasses of milk.

In other words, I would have been full.

We went to a restaurant in the same village and ordered crepes. I should say "crepe" singular. They only brought one on a plate. My husband and I stared at our respective "dinners" and wondered how they got away with charging ten Euros for a single pancake.

For a moment I thought it was a comment on our American girth, although neither of us fell into the BMI overweight category. I glanced around. We weren't the only ones punished with meager portions. In fact, the other diners seemed to enjoy eating their dinners, taking small bites, enjoying them, seemingly in no hurry. They were conversing more than they were eating.

We shrugged and agreed, "When in Rome . . . ."

To our surprise, we weren't hungry when we finished our crepe. We were satisfied. My husband didn't ask for another helping. Or a refund.

After a few days of this, we recognized something we usually hadn't before. Instead of eating until we felt full (stuffed, to be blunt), we stopped when our stomachs sent us signals that they were satiated.

⹌ 19 ⹌

What Is Satiety?

SATIETY IS THE TERM used by dietitians to mean fullness or satisfaction—a sense of adequate food consumption. It originates in the thousands of sensors that line our stomach wall, but it's a delicate signal with a delay.

Most of the sensors we interact with provide immediate feedback. We walk toward a door, and it automatically opens fast enough for us to enter. We put our hands near the faucet in the bathroom, and water flows. We swipe our credit cards, and the machine immediately tells me we've maxed out our credit. (If only they could program it with "junk food credit" instead of counting all purchases equally!)

Being hungry isn't like an on/off switch. The biological sensors in our stomachs are more sophisticated; they respond to physics, gravity, chemistry, and geometry to tell our hypothalamus that we're hungry. Like an air conditioner's thermostat, our stomach sensors operate in a gradual fashion. In our condo in the winter, I often find myself getting cold. Just as I get up to check if the heater is working, it kicks in. Then it gets a little too hot before it shuts off.

So most of the time, I'm just a little too cool or too warm.

My husband likes to quote a poem his grandfather recited all the time:

As a rule, man's a fool.
When it's hot, he wants it cool.
When it's cool, he wants it hot.
Always wanting what is not.

Our stomachs are like that. As they empty, the sensors start accumulating data, building toward a trigger point. Then they send a tentative signal to the brain: time to start thinking about finding food. A little later, they send more signals: any chance there's food out there somewhere? Then more sensors kick in: okay, now we're serious—we'd like you to eat something. If we ignore the signals, they get more insistent. Whatever you're doing, stop. It's time to eat.

The stomach sensors can get downright obnoxious the longer you ignore them.

So then we respond. Like the heater coming on, we provide relief by eating something. Once we get started, we keep going.

The sensors respond: Hey, thanks. We're good.

In my condo, I'm thinking, I'm just about right. But the heater keeps blowing hot air.

And we keep eating.

The stomach is starting to expand. The chemical and physical sensors are sending more messages, but we ignore them. We have a plate to clean here, guys. Leave us alone.

The little metal coil in the heater's thermostat is expanding, but it's not quite there, so the heater keeps pumping out the hot air.

And we keep eating.

Then, finally, the thermostat trips. The gas valve shuts off, the flames stop burning, the fan stops blowing, and I'm not getting any hotter. Finally.

And we've reached a point where we can't take another bite. We're stuffed. Actually, we're uncomfortable. Maybe we're mad at ourselves. Maybe our stomachs are painful and bloated. We might feel guilt or discouragement. Some of us might get depressed. In extreme cases, we can experience self-loathing.

Let's back up a minute and see what happened.

The sensation of physical emptiness builds gradually until it becomes a powerful biological hunger that we can't ignore. The sensation of satiety also builds gradually until it produces that stuffed, uncomfortable feeling.

But just as we can calibrate a heater's thermostat, we can learn to calibrate our own responses to our stomach's sensors.

— 20 —

Calibrating Physical Fullness

IF WE CAN retrain ourselves to recognize true stomach hunger we can feed our physical hunger—the sensation of emptiness—more effectively without overeating.

How did we get trained in the first place?

Any parent who has cooked a meal hates to see the effort wasted. Back when families ate meals together, we told our kids something like this: "Clear your plate before you can be excused." Now, it's more like, "You better eat all that stuff I bought at McDonald's."

Either way, the lesson we're teaching is to eat based on external signals. It's not what your stomach is telling you but it's what on your plate (or in the McDonald's wrapper).

And that's exactly the wrong signal in a country where 96% of restaurant entrees exceed USDA limits for calories, sodium, fat and saturated fat.[30]

Our experience in France was typical of our food experiences around the world. In Mumbai, India, I ordered a Masala Dosa that cost less than a dollar. It was essentially a paper-thin crispy pancake (sort of a thin crepe) with a filling of spicy legumes that was about three tablespoons. It was the ideal size for giving me satiety but not supersatiety. In Thailand, the entrees are about half the size they are in American Thai restaurants.

---

30. Wu & Sturm (2012) "What's on the menu? A review of the energy and nutritional content of U.S. chain restaurant menus," *Public Health Nutrition,* May 11, 2012:1-10

It takes practice and conscious effort to concentrate on stomach sensations to become aware of our satiety level. We have a lot to overcome; most of us are desensitized to our stomach's sensors. One study showed that when certain mice are fed a steady diet of saturated fat, they become less sensitive to leptin (the hormone that suppresses appetite) and insulin.[31] The rats ignored the satiety signals from the stomach. Whether humans are similarly affected is not clear, but we do ignore our satiety signals when we don't wait for them to kick in (eat too fast) or when we eat what's in front of us (clear our plate) regardless of how we feel.

Books such as *Eating Awareness Training* by Molly Groger advocate exercises to focus on a point in the center of your abdomen, become aware of the sensation, and rate your hunger.[32] Instead of Ms. Groger's 10-point scale, a one-to-five scale works more quickly to check on your hand. One is extremely hungry and five is extremely full. Three is neutral and comfortable. Two is hungry, time to refill. Four is full, you've had enough.

---

31. Benoit et al, (2009) Palmitic acid mediates hypothalamic insulin resistance, The Journal of Clinical Investigation, 119:9
32. Groger, M. & Lebherz, T. (1985) *Eating Awareness Training: The Natural Way to Permanent Weight Loss* Simon & Schuster, New York

Five-Point Hunger Scale

5	**Way overfull and very uncomfortable** (You ate too much and regret it, may be in pain)
4.5	(A little too full, uncomfortable)
4	**Full, just finished eating enough** (Conscious that you have had enough to eat)
3.5	(Starting to feel full)
3	**Neutral, comfortable** (Not interested in eating and not overfull)
2.5	(Only slightly hungry)
2	**Hungry** (Conscious of needing to eat, time to refill)
1.5	(Very hungry)
1	**Extremely hungry, "starving!"** (You waited too long to eat, now feeling deprived)

To help assign a rating, you can imagine drinking a quart of milk or water. Do you feel that empty? (You're at 2 or lower.) Or does the idea bring a slight gag reflex? (You might be 3 or higher.)

Could you eat an entire apple? (You're at 2 or lower.) Or is it more like a single slice your stomach wants? (Maybe 2.5 or higher.) Imagine your stomach as a balloon and visualize how big it is. Is it stretching? (About 4.5.) Is it about to pop? (You may be at 5.)

You can also use a tracker or food journal to help you keep

track of your hunger score at different points of the day. Start when you first wake up, and then take readings in the morning, mid-morning, noon, afternoon, evening, and bedtime. At each point make observations and discern patterns. Soon you'll notice sensations that lead to conclusions such as these:

In the mid-morning if you are at 3 you are probably not hungry but just eating out of habit.

At noon if you are at 2.5, you are really only slightly hungry, maybe just reacting to the cue of the clock. But at 1:00 p.m. if you are at 2, you know you are hungry and need to eat before you start feeling really deprived.

If you note that by 5:00 p.m. you are always at level 2 or even 1.5, you may decide to have an early dinner or you will need at least a snack instead of waiting until 8:00 p.m. for your normal time to eat dinner.

Test yourself for a few days or a week and you'll see how you can calibrate your stomach sensors. Once you recognize the feeling of satiety that comes with eating smaller portions over a longer period of time, you'll look forward to mealtime and avoid the discomfort and guilt associated with overeating.

21

What Is Energy Density?

BEFORE WE VISITED Antarctica, my husband talked to a man who was assigned to Antarctica in the Russian Navy. He wondered why my husband wanted to visit Antarctica, as if one would be crazy to *voluntarily* go.

"I want to see the penguins," my husband said.

"I hate penguins," the Russian said, waving his hand in disgust.

"How could anyone hate penguins?"

The Russian shook his head. "That's all we had to eat for six months!"

Now that I've been to Antarctica and visited the penguin colonies, I have a better appreciation for what my husband's Russian friend said. The penguins are smelly. I imagine they'd taste like fish, except greasy and tough. But it made sense for the Russian Navy to use them for food. You need a lot of calories to survive in Antarctica, and penguin meat is energy dense.

I'm not advocating penguin meat (they have enough problems avoiding leopard seals and coping with climate change), but I do want you to consider energy density in your choice of foods. Unless you're living in Antarctica or you're a professional athlete, you probably aren't suffering from a lack of calories. But you are probably eating energy dense food more than you realize.

The concept of energy density helps identify the satiety contributions of foods. Energy density means calories per mass.

Strawberries, for example, have few calories in comparison to their mass. By contrast, a candy bar with the same mass (or bulk) has many times the calorie content.

Think of the difference in terms of your choices. If you want a snack, strawberries (low energy density) will fill you up when a candy bar won't. You can eat 4 ½ cups of strawberries that contain the same calories as a 1½ ounce bar of chocolate that your stomach will hardly notice. You don't even want to know how many calories of chocolate it would take to fill 4 ½ cups, do you?

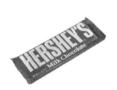 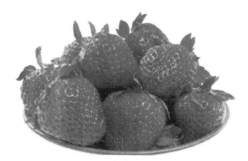

1.5 oz bar   OR   4.5 cups fruit
220 calories   220 calories

High energy density food is high in calories but low in mass. Low energy density food has more bulk and fewer calories. As a general rule, you will feel fuller eating low energy dense foods because they put pressure on the satiety sensors of the stomach, without excess calories.

Highest in energy density are the foods we call "empty calories" because they supply calories but provide little bulk for the satiety sensors. Such foods include anything high in fat or sugar, fried foods, refined white flour, and heavily sweetened foods.

In my view, the most insidious high energy dense food is the soft drink. Their liquid form makes them elusive to the satiety sensors of the stomach, so you can drink great quantities without feeling full.

Foods high in sugar are a hunger paradox. As simple carbs, they satisfy the Sweet Sally Syndrome, the craving stemming from low blood sugar. But being energy dense, they do not trigger the satiety sensors. We miseat because we're eating lots of sugar but we remain hungry.

The great advantage to low energy dense foods is that we feel full without overdoing our calorie intake. As expressed in the vintage Grape Nuts slogan, a low energy dense food *"fills you up but not out."*

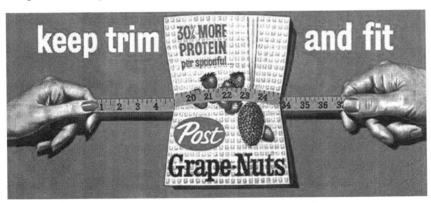

22

What Is Nutrient Density?

THERE'S ANOTHER ASPECT of penguin meat that the Russian Navy and leopard seals know instinctively but probably couldn't articulate -- nutrient density.

Instead of just measuring volume and calories, *nutrient density* measures how much of a nutrient is supplied per calorie of food. This could be measured for any nutrient, i.e., the Vitamin C density of oranges is higher than the Vitamin C density of bread.

We usually focus on nutrient density in terms of nutrients that are in short supply in an average diet. For example, the nutrient density for fiber would compare how much fiber per calorie in different foods. Oatmeal has high fiber density, but refined foods have low fiber density (if any).

We hear a lot in the media about processed foods. It's not that processing is inherently bad; food processing has made possible abundant, inexpensive foods throughout the world and is a major factor in the elimination of hunger and nutritional disorders in developing countries. However, we have to make informed choices.

Consider the apple. An apple off the tree has high fiber density. Take that same apple and process it into sweetened apple sauce; you've lost fiber density. Process it some more, turning it into apple juice, and you've lost essentially all the fiber.

The same thing happens with grains. Compare raw wheat to white flour, for example. Check for this the next time you buy bread.

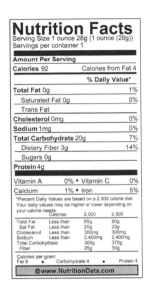

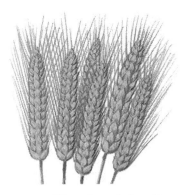

Wheat in grain form[27]

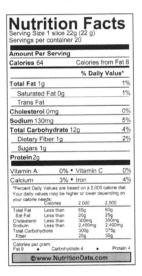

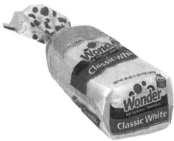

Refined white bread[28]

Refined white bread

An example of Vitamin E density: you would need only one slice of wheat bread to get the same amount of Vitamin E as five slices of white bread. In other words, if your food is higher in nutrients you would need a lot less to meet your body's needs.

Another example demonstrates the fiber density in two cereals. Even though oatmeal is higher in calories than Rice Krispies, oatmeal

---

33. Nutritional data and wheat label image courtesy of www.NutritionData.com
34. Bread label and bread label image courtesy of www.wonderbread.com/

has ten times the fiber per calorie, so it will supply a lot more for the body—higher satiety, longer lasting, and more nutritious.

Fiber Density

Oatmeal

- ▸ 166 calories
- ▸ 4 grams fiber
- ▸ ND = 24 mg/cal
- ▸ *10 times the fiber/cal*

Rice Krispies

128 calories ◂
0.3 grams fiber ◂
ND = 2.3 mg/cal ◂

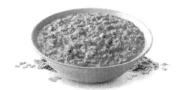
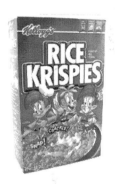

Our foods have a great variety of nutrients so one single measure cannot evaluate the complexities of what we need. One way to evaluate foods is to integrate values for several vitamins and minerals at once with an aggregate nutrient density score.

Dr. Joel Fuhrman developed the Nutrient Density Line,[35] representing one way to compare the relative contribution of foods. Dr. Fuhrman studied a long list of nutrients to see how many beneficial items foods contribute compared to their calorie content. He ranks vegetables as having the highest nutrient density scores, followed by beans and fruits, then seeds and nuts, whole grains and potatoes. Lowest are sweets and processed foods.

---

35. Fuhrman, J. *Nutrient Density*, available at http://www.drfuhrman.com/library/article17.aspx

A similar index is documented on the *Eat Right America* Web site,[36] where a table is provided of sixty-six common foods, each analyzed for the aggregate list of identified nutrients.

You can see more details on their Web site, but here is a sample of their nutrient density scores.

Kale	100	Apple	7	White Bread	2
Broccoli	37	Peas	7	Cheese	2
Carrots	24	Oatmeal	5	Potato Chips	1
Strawberries	21	Cucumber	5	Ice Cream	1
Tomato	16	Salmon	4	French Fries	1
Blueberries	13	Avocado	4	Cola	0

Again the highest scores come from fruits and vegetables. Kale's score of 100 means it supplies more of all the nutrients for less calories than all the other foods. Lowest scores come from foods with too many calories compared to the limited number of nutrients provided. The lowest score of all is cola which suggests it has empty calories and nothing else to recommend it.

36. http://www.eatrightamerica.com/erni-superfoods

23

Suggestions for Greater Satiety

OUR SATIETY THERMOSTAT is the second stealth hunger that misleads us into poor eating habits if we let it. The satiety sensors operate on the volume of food in our stomachs. Like the heaters in our homes, the sensors work gradually. If we're not sensitive to them, we won't eat until they've set off a five-alarm signal. Then, if we don't eat slowly or if we eat in response to an external stimulus such as the amount of food on our plate or the portion served at the restaurant, we don't give our sensors time to respond and we overeat.

Our sensors are, ultimately, not that smart. They don't care whether the food is energy or nutrient dense. If it has volume, the sensors will detect it, end of story. Satiety is the easiest of the stealth appetites to feed; even food that will not raise our blood sugar (see Part 1) will still fill up the stomach and create that feeling of being done.

If we fill our stomachs with penguin meat or chocolate or whole-wheat bread, our satiety sensors will give the same signal based on the volume of the food. So we want to watch not only how much we eat, and how we eat it, but what we eat.

High Satiety Foods

A study done in Australia demonstrated how different foods create various levels of satiety.[37] Dr. Susanna Holt gave people

---

37. Holt, S.H.A., et al (1995) A satiety index of common foods, European Journal of Clinical Nutrition, 49: 675-690

different foods, but always the same number of calories (240 cal) and measured how long they felt full. They used a slice of white bread as the standard, and called it 100% satiety. Other foods were assigned a different score showing how full the subjects were.

Satiety Index
240 calories

Donut	White Bread	French Fries	Oatmeal	Boiled Potatoes
68%	100%	116%	209%	323%

Susanna Holt, PhD: European Journal of Clinical Nutrition

A doughnut received a score of only 68%, meaning that after eating it they felt full for only 68% as long as the white bread made them full. A bowl of oatmeal with the same calories got a score of 209%, meaning it kept them full over twice as long as the bread.

Some other interesting values were 116% for French fries, but 323% for the same number of calories from boiled potatoes, which were the highest satiety-producing foods in their study. Other conclusions about what works for satiety:

- Whole grain breads give higher satiety than white

- High fiber increases satiety

- High fat decreases satiety

- Cakes, doughnuts and croissants gave lower satiety

- Fruits and vegetables gave higher satiety.

FingerTIPS about Physical Emptiness

- Rate your physical hunger by concentrating on a point in the center of your abdomen and assign a value between 1 and 5.

- When your stomach signals true hunger, look for low energy density foods to fill it.

- Eat slowly to give your brain time to receive the satiety signals from your stomach.

- In choosing foods, consider the nutrient density of your choices to make sure you are giving your body the best advantages possible.

- If you still feel like eating when your stomach gives signals that it has reached satiety, discover other hungers you may be experiencing (see Parts 3, 4, and 5).

Resources about Physical Emptiness

FOLLOWING ARE SOME helpful books and articles to explore for more information as you become more aware of the second hunger.

Rolls, Barbara (2012) *The Ultimate Volumetrics Diet: Smart, Simple, Science-Based Strategies for Losing Weight and Keeping It Off*, Harper Collins: New York

> Suggests eating plans based on low energy density so you can fill up on more foods.

Ornish, Dean (2000) *Eat More, Weigh Less: Dr. Dean Ornish's Life Choice Program for Losing Weight Safely While Eating Abundantly*, Harper Collins: New York

> Takes the approach of abundance rather than deprivation to lose weight and reduce risk for cancer and other chronic diseases.

Nutritiondata.com, *The Fullness Factor* Available at http://nutritiondata.self.com/topics/fullness-factor

> Gives a predicted level of satiety to common foods based on a mathematical formula and the ingredient content.

Zinczenko, David and Goulding, Matt, (2011) Eat This, Not That! *The No-Diet Weight Loss Solution*. Rodale: New York

> Editors of *Men's Health* magazine distill diet decisions down to simple comparisons between foods with high energy density compared to better choices, with colorful photos of common fast food meals and favorite foods.

Groger, M. & Lebherz, T. (1985) *Eating Awareness Training: The Natural Way to Permanent Weight Loss,* Simon & Schuster: New York

> Presents a six-week program to teach awareness of when your body has enough, protect yourself from an unhealthy urge to eat, and be free from diets and calorie counting.

26

FingerFOODS
Recipe for the Second Hunger

HELP FILL YOUR empty stomach with this alternative to a traditional favorite. Veggie spaghetti has both lower energy density and higher nutrient density than regular spaghetti pasta. This means you will be fuller on less food, and you will meet more of your body's nutritional needs at the same time.

Veggie Spaghetti has something for everyone: very low carb, gluten-free, high potassium . . . and the mild flavor fits in well with any traditional spaghetti sauce.

Veggie Spaghetti

1 medium spaghetti squash (cucurbita pepo)
4 cups marinara sauce, canned, bottled or made fresh
1 onion, chopped
1 cup mushrooms, diced
1 Tbsp olive oil
2 Tbsp grated parmesan cheese

Cut the squash in half and remove seeds.
Cook by roasting 30 to 40 minutes at 375° or boiling/
steaming about 20 minutes. Best texture comes from being
careful not to overcook. Squash is done when the strands
separate easily with a fork. Sauté onions and mushrooms
in olive oil and stir in marinara sauce. Serve over strands of
squash. Top with Parmesan cheese.

Makes 8 servings of 1 cup squash and ½ cup sauce.

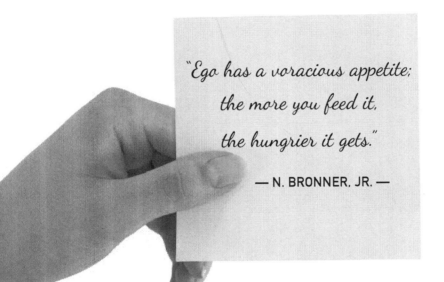

"Ego has a voracious appetite;
the more you feed it,
the hungrier it gets."

— N. BRONNER, JR. —

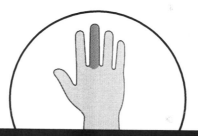

÷ PART III ÷

The Middle Finger

The Third Hunger Is Emotional Emptiness

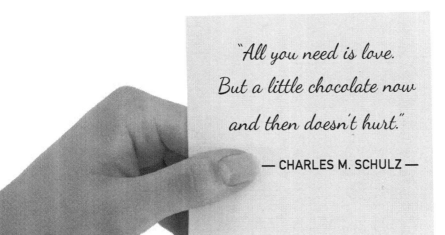

"All you need is love.
But a little chocolate now
and then doesn't hurt."

— CHARLES M. SCHULZ —

27

"... I've Hungered for Your Touch ..."

ONE OF THE MOST recorded songs of the last century, "Unchained Melody," was written in 1955, made famous by the Righteous Brothers in 1965, and then received new acclaim in the blockbuster 1990 film *Ghost*. Its popularity stems in part from the universal and haunting lyrics, sung as the ghost of Patrick Swayze reaches for his still-living wife, Demi Moore:

"Oh, my love, my darling, I've hungered for your touch, a long lonely time."

The ghost's inability to actually touch the living human contrasted with Moore's shaping of pottery, a highly physical activity. Audiences felt the anguish of unfulfilled longing because we've all felt such longing in our own lives (setting aside the ghost aspect).

The stealth appetite of emotional emptiness is a universal human experience. Poetry and philosophy use *hunger* as a metaphor for mental, emotional, or spiritual emptiness. But emotional hunger is not merely a metaphor; it's a very real, physical feeling that is easy to confuse with physical hunger.

Many different feelings can be misinterpreted as physical hunger. Some are obvious parallels to stomach emptiness, such as loneliness or the grief of loss, where a vague sensation that something or someone is missing feels very much like physical hunger and triggers the instinct to replenish food missing from the stomach.

Almost any emotion can create a desire or longing that can be confused with physical hunger. It's not always negative, either. People stock up on junk food for Super Bowl Weekend because the excitement makes us feel hungry. But more commonly, sadness, boredom, anxiety, and anger create an emotional turmoil that demands resolution. The brain seeks to calm these unpleasant sensations. Remembering from many years of reinforcement that food comforts and rewards, the brain naturally recommends a food remedy.

The highly pleasurable sensations of taste and chewing have reinforced this response so that it is a strong instinct to reach for food to calm emotional distress. This one mechanism is a major reason people have trouble following through with healthy intentions. No other response has as immediate or as strong an effect as food does to blunt the feeling of emptiness.

In this way human beings are different from animals: we eat not only to feed our bodies but also to satisfy other non-physical hungers.

This isn't just an American problem, either.

Grace Makutsi, a character created by Alexander McCall Smith, is a delightful woman living in Botswana. In one story[38] she has been excitedly expecting the delivery of a beautiful bed. When it will not fit through the door and she realizes she will not get the new bed after all, she is devastated. Wondering what to do next, she finally decides to just go out and buy doughnuts.

Grace is demonstrating how she feels acutely the lack of the anticipated new furniture and knows that absence can be temporarily filled with doughnuts. It is human nature to turn to food to fill up our emptiness.

---

38. McCall Smith, A. (2009) *The Miracle at Speedy Motors*, A No. 1 Ladies' Detective Agency Novel, Random House

28

The Supermarket as Pharmacy

THE SUPERMARKET AISLES in America are falsely labeled. I was at a store recently and saw a sign overhead that read: Cookies, Snacks. Another sign read: Soft Drinks, Beer. A third read: Candy, Chips.

The signs should have read: Happiness! Serenity! Friends! Self-Confidence! Excitement!

Because what are those foods, really? They're not high in beneficial nutrients. We've seen they don't satisfy stealth appetite #1; Sweet Sally Syndrome thrives on these products. They don't satisfy stealth appetite #2, either; in fact, they are so energy dense you'd have to eat a days' worth of calories in one sitting to feel full.

But there has to be a justification for their placement in our supermarkets. And there is.

Except they belong in the pharmacy department, not the food aisles.

These "foods" are often used as cures for depression, anxiety, loneliness, and boredom. You should treat them as an extension of the pharmacy.

How much time do you spend in the aisles comparing aspirin to Motrin? That's how much time you should spend buying candy and chips and soft drinks.

I'm not saying these "foods" are bad, any more than aspirin is bad. They're not. They have their place. But most of the time when we consume them, we don't realize we're succumbing to the stealth appetite #3: emotional emptiness.

I worked with patients suffering from anorexia, bulimia, and compulsive overeating in an Eating Disorders program in California. Our patients had traumatic emotional needs underlying their food obsessions. Years earlier, Nancy had been in a devastating car collision that killed her daughter. Nancy not only missed her daughter terribly, but she felt responsible for her death and could not forgive herself. Ever since that tragedy, Nancy described herself as a compulsive over eater. She used food to console herself and blunt the painful guilt and regret.

Other eating disorder patients had different stories but all were painful and emotional. Some had been molested, others had lost a spouse or child, and many had done things they regretted terribly. All had learned that food worked as a temporary coping mechanism. And they were in treatment because their disordered eating (extreme *miseating*) had reached the point of interfering with daily functioning. These were dramatic cases, but they had similarities to each of us and our occasional episodes of using food to calm ourselves.

Without realizing it, we are using food for self-medication, and then suffering the side effects.

What if we decided we didn't need doctors and pharmacists anymore? Anyone could buy any medication, for any reason. It would be up to us to decide how much of what medications to take for what symptoms—or no symptoms at all, as long as the drugs made us feel better.

The idea of medicating ourselves with wild abandon is preposterous, but we do the same thing with food.

Those "comfort food" aisles are the equivalent of candy-flavored kids' aspirin, but without the child-proof caps. Side effects include high blood pressure, obesity, and death.

And it's not only the "junk food" aisles. Any food can be a

comfort food if it makes us feel better emotionally. I've had clients who stayed away from cookies and candy but binged on pot pies or frozen waffles. I've seen peanut butter obsession, pizza obsession, and cold cereal obsession.

There are plenty of books (and therapists) who address the deeper psychological issues. I've found that even well-educated, sensible, and otherwise healthy people like you and me don't recognize the stealth hunger of emotional emptiness.

Try this exercise: next time you walk down one of the junk food aisles, ask yourself what you're feeling.

Are you low in blood sugar, Sweet Sally? Walk over to the fresh fruit section.

Are you feeling hungry because your stomach sensors are beeping? Go get some vegetables and whole grain bread.

Are you upset or angry? Lonely? Bored? Then maybe you've come to the right place, but remember, you're in *an unregulated pharmacy*, not a food store.

Choose wisely.

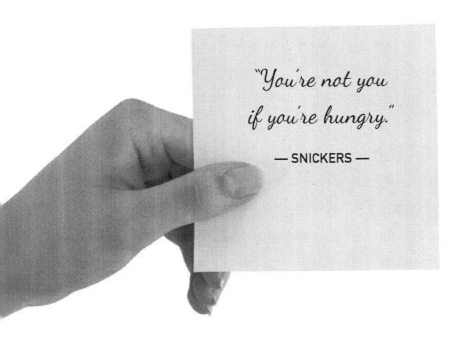

"You're not you
if you're hungry."

— SNICKERS —

29

Healthy Food at Celebrations

I HAVE BEEN teaching a college nutrition course for many years. Each class is different, and sometimes a particular class stands out for better or worse. Last year I had a large enthusiastic evening class, and the students enjoyed learning how to make healthier choices and improve their personal nutrition. They asked if we could plan a big party for the last night of class, and several students volunteered to bring food. I was excited to anticipate how they would demonstrate what they had learned by bringing healthy alternatives to the party.

That night I came thirty minutes early to set up, only to find that the students had already brought their food contributions: a large plate of glazed donuts, a large chocolate cake, and several 2-liter bottles of soft drinks. I asked the woman who had organized the pot-luck, "But what about some healthy choices?" She looked just as perplexed as I was and replied, "What do you mean? This is a party!"

Although we had talked for hours in class about healthy eating, she still believed that to celebrate or have a treat, the food had to be decadent -- high in fat and high in sugar. To her, it couldn't be a party without "forbidden" foods that you would then feel guilty about consuming.

I still had time to dash out and buy a large vegetable platter, some cut fruit, and a bag of clementines (small tangerines), which I quietly added to the food table before class started.

As the students filed into class, they filled up their food plates.

Four or five of them made remarks like, "thanks for including some healthy food" and "I was expecting I would not be able to eat anything because I'm trying to cut back on sweets." At the end of class we packed up the leftovers. I was gratified to see that the vegetable tray was cleaned off and most of the fruit had been eaten. The cake and donuts in contrast had been only lightly sampled. Somehow, the students had incorporated the nutrition principles we had discussed.

Like the student who couldn't imagine a party without gooey treats, many of us don't realize that even celebrations can be healthy and nourishing. At your next birthday party, family gathering, or church or community social, challenge yourself to remember the healthy alternatives. Do a favor to those who are trying to develop healthier eating habits and make the menu colorful, healthy, and guilt-free with this simple rule:

The best desserts are fruits, and the best snacks are vegetables.

You can even decorate with their natural colors.

Nothing is as colorful as fresh raw vegetables, which could include cucumbers, carrots, cherry tomatoes and sweet bell peppers in red, orange, yellow and green. A fruit platter becomes automatically festive with contrasting colors such as red strawberries surrounding green grapes, or blueberries garnishing a tray of watermelon and pineapple chunks.

Both fruits and vegetables offer an outlet for your artistic abilities, for carving and decorating. You can see amazing examples with a simple internet search for fruit and vegetable carving.[39]

---

39. For a start, see http://www.fruitcarving.com/ and http://www.foodgarnishing.com/id27.html

30

Side Effects

I CONFESS, I have my own "comfort foods." I like to make Rice Krispie treats with marshmallows. I like mashed potatoes. And I like ice cream whenever possible. Because I'm always thinking in terms of the five hungers, I recognize that I'm not really craving sugar, and my stomach isn't empty when I eat these things.

I'm responding to my emotional hunger.

As with all the hungers, there is a continuum between disinterest and "gotta have it!" Setting aside for now the effectiveness of food to satisfy emotional hunger, I want to discuss the side effects.

When I worked with serious eating disorders in a clinical setting, the side effects were obvious. People were aggravating their emotional hungers by feeding them. They were *miseating*.

What about the far more common emotional hungers we've all experienced? Are there side effects from self-medicating our occasional bouts of anxiety or stress with food?

First, the "calming medication" effect we get from food is temporary and needs constant replenishment. Secondly, responding to emotional stimuli makes us fill our stomachs with more food than our system can use, and our organs have to work overtime to process the unnecessary nutrients. Weight gain is the most frequent side effect. In turn this can cause emotional distress, often worse than the original needs it was meant to satisfy.

Here are some other ways people fill their emptiness with food:

George just broke up with his girlfriend. As he faces ordinary daily routines he used to share with her, he has a sense that something is missing, which feels like hunger. Eating satisfies the hunger but the satisfaction does not last. As he continues to renew the comfort factor by eating more, the sense of loss might be diminished momentarily, but George begins to establish habits of overeating that become permanent and can lead to chronic disease.

Marlene longs to look like the slim models presented by TV and movies as the ideal. The longing for this unmet goal creates a sense of emptiness, which feels a lot like hunger. She receives a temporary easing of the hunger by eating. However, in one to three hours the momentary satisfaction is gone. As she realizes she is no closer to her ideal image, the hunger returns and she wants to eat again. As she continues to *miseat*, she gains weight and her reality grows farther away from her ideal image.

31

Research on Emotional Eating

EMOTIONAL EATING responds to one of the strongest of all hungers. In a 2003 study, researchers noted how brain circuits have the potential to be affected by natural rewards like food.[40] The sensitivity of the brain to these natural rewards is "correlated positively with measures of emotional overeating."[41]

Another study, by Dr. Lukas Van Oudenhove, demonstrated how sad emotions may be soothed by fatty foods.[42] After inducing sad emotions in test subjects through musical and visual cues, researchers then injected fatty acids into subjects' stomachs and noted how these sad emotions were lessened by the fatty acid infusion. The study ultimately highlighted the interplay between food, emotions, hunger, food intake, and meal-induced sensations in health.

Our moods and emotions clearly affect our food intake. One study looked at the amount of food eaten during positive and negative moods, then amounts eaten alone compared to what was eaten in social situations.[43]

---

40. Davis, C., Strachan, S., Berkson, M. (2004) "Sensitivity to reward: implications for overeating and overweight," Appetite, 42 (2) 131-138

41. Ibid

42. Van Oudenhove, L. et al, (2011) " Fatty acid–induced gut-brain signaling attenuates neural and behavioral effects of sad emotion in humans," Journal of Clinical Investigation.121(8):3094–3099

43. Patel, K.A., & Schlundt, D.G. (2001) "Impact of Moods and Social Context on Eating Behavior, *Appetite*, 36(2) p 111-118

Results showed that food intake increased during both positive and negative moods compared to amounts eaten when in a neutral mood. When people were in a social situation, meals were significantly larger, regardless of mood.

The important message is that our emotions have a very real impact on eating. When we acknowledge that, we can anticipate emotional cues and social situations and plan ahead for how we want to respond.

+ 32 +

Distinguish Physical from Emotional Hunger

PATRICK SWAYZE's ghost knew the difference between physical and emotional emptiness. A ghost (presumably) can't have physical hunger; there are no "empty" signals from a stomach to a brain and in any case, no food to fill the stomach if there were. But the ghost's emotional hunger was intense.

Because we're alive, we have an advantage over ghosts. We can learn to recognize the difference between physical and emotional emptiness and find alternative ways to feed our emotional hungers besides *miseating*.

Understanding emotional emptiness starts first by concentrating on our physical sensations (as discussed in Part 2) before identifying when the emptiness is from physical hunger and when it is emotional.

When I encouraged people to check their physical fullness with a satiety rating of one to five (see Chapter 20), they often told me they had usually reached for food automatically without even thinking if they were hungry or not. It is similar with emotional hungers and very common to be somewhat oblivious to what we are longing for or worrying about.

If you have assessed your physical hunger and decided your rating is at 3 or more, but you still want to eat, it helps to then assess your emotional hunger.

Emotional Hunger Checklist

- ⬛ Have you suffered the recent loss of a friend, family member, or pet?

- ⬛ Are you missing someone who is absent (even temporarily)?

- ⬛ Has a project that was absorbing your attention recently ended?

- ⬛ Are you feeling left out of someone else's plans?

- ⬛ Were you passed over for an award, privilege, or recognition?

- ⬛ Do you know someone in need whom you wish you could help but are unable to do anything?

- ⬛ Do you think someone else is disappointed in you?

- ⬛ Are you nervous about something you have to do in the future?

- ⬛ Are you tired of a current situation and wish it were over?

- ⬛ Are you worried about the results of a recent effort, application, or test?

- ⬛ Do you have any other unmet emotional need?

With the checklist you can run through several emotional cues that might be reminding you of food. After completing the Emotional Hunger Checklist either mentally or on paper, you can acknowledge your emotional needs and decide the best way to handle them.

The checklist can be the start of your record-keeping, to begin to track feelings in the food journals included at the end of this chapter.

Don't Forget to Consider Stress

Some people who *miseat* need stress management skills more than they need diet advice, because stress is a major cause of overeating. Researchers at Harvard have noted how stress hormones increase appetite and may also ramp up motivation in general, including the motivation to eat: [44]

> [...] Fat- and sugar-filled foods seem to have a feedback effect that inhibits activity in the parts of the brain that produce and process stress and related emotions. These foods really are "comfort" foods in that they seem to counteract stress—and this may contribute to people's stress-induced craving for those foods.

Of course, *miseating* in turn can increase other stress, especially if a person has felt frustrated about attempts to control eating. The response to this stress can lead to a discouraging, vicious cycle. Remember as you assess your hungers to also look at the stressors (what is causing you stress) and what you are doing to deal with stress.

---

44. Harvard Mental Health Letter, "Why stress causes people to overeat" February 2012, available at http://www.health.harvard.edu/newsletters/Harvard_Mental_Health_Letter/2012/February/why-stress-causes-people-to-overeat

Stop and think about the factors in your life that add to your burden of stress. Be sure to consider whether you may be reacting to your stress by *miseating*.

Many excellent guides are available that offer tips on healthy stress management. Because stress is known to be one significant risk factor for heart disease, the American Heart Association provides stress management tools such as *Fight Stress with Healthy Habits*.[45]

Food Journals

The first step in managing your emotional eating is to keep a food journal, sometimes called a *tracker*, to record when you eat, how much, and why.

You can design your own version of a food tracker or journal, according to the information you want to know about your hungers. Microsoft Office even supplies several templates for food diaries as Word documents or Excel spreadsheets you can customize.[46]

On the next page are some simplified examples you can modify to suit your own situation, and transfer to larger sheets.

---

45. Available at http://www.heart.org/HEARTORG/GettingHealthy/StressManagement/ FightStressWithHealthyHabits/Fight-Stress-with-Healthy-Habits_UCM_307992_ Article.jsp

46. Available at office.microsoft.com/en-us/templates/food-diary-TC006089420.aspx

Foods	Amount	When	Where	Why Which finger/ Which hunger?
1.				
2.				
3.				
4.				
5.				
6.				
Etc.				

Foods	Time	Feelings Before Eating	Feelings After Eating	Which finger/ Which hunger?
1.				
2.				
3.				
4.				
5.				
6.				
Etc.				

Time	Foods	Meal or Snack?	Reason for Eating Which finger/ Which hunger?
6:00 a.m.			
7:00 a.m.			
8:00 a.m.			
9:00 a.m.			
10:00 a.m.			
11:00 a.m.			
Etc.			

Find Ways to Fill Emotional Emptiness

EMOTIONS ARE A wonderful and amazing part of life and are unique to each individual. As you become more aware of your own emotional reactions and how you turn to certain foods in response to certain feelings, you will learn what works for you. Your own uniquely personal strategies will help you avoid unwanted side effects from the "self-medication."

As you recognize your emotional eating behavior with a food tracker or journal, you will need alternative ways to feed those emotions. Plan rewarding non-food distractions to help calm yourself. With the money you would have spent on comfort foods, buy yourself something with fewer side effects than miseating brings you.

There are three main categories of alternatives to miseating for emotional reasons. Each feeds a different type of emotion. The effectiveness of each will depend on your particular mood at the time, as well as your personality and social setting, but consider trying each one to give you the broadest range of satisfying emotions to fill the emotional holes.

1. Intellectual stimulation: hobbies, reading, puzzles, mental challenges

2. Physical activities: recreation, sports, exercises, walking, or simply enjoying nature

3. Giving service: concentrating on filling another's needs through community, church, or other voluntary activity

All of these help bring emotional satisfaction that compensates for emotional emptiness. That emotional satisfaction feels a lot like satiety or fullness—but without the side effects.

Intellectual Stimulation

People have sought intellectual stimulation from the beginning of recorded history. Chess, for example, was first played 1500 years ago. Boards and pieces for the precursor of checkers have been found in digs as old as 600 BC in Egypt.

Now there are many types of mental puzzles and games we can play as individuals, as well. Do you like numbers and adding in your head? You will probably enjoy Sudoku and Kakuro. Are you more verbal? You might like crossword puzzles and word games.

Reward yourself and take care of your emotional needs with a new book by your favorite author, or a fresh new book of crossword puzzles, or an electronic Sudoku game.

Even trying a new recipe, such as the ones in this book, can prove intellectually stimulating!

Physical Activity

Researchers such as Dr. John Ratey, professor of psychiatry at Harvard Medical School, report that physical exercise can have remarkable effects on emotional and mental states. In his recent book,[47] Dr. Ratey explores the connection between what your body does and what your mind feels. He presents evidence that exercise helps prevent depression, addiction, aggression, and Alzheimer's.

47. Ratey, J. (2008) Spark: *The Revolutionary New Science of Exercise and the Brain*, Little, Brown and Company, New York

The importance of exercise is not a new discovery. Decades ago sports physiologists such as John Raglin[48] found an association between exercise and improved mood. His research showed that after 20 to 40 minutes of aerobic exercise, anxiety was decreased and mood was improved for several hours, and even more pronounced effects were seen on those who started with elevated anxiety or depression. He also cautioned that moderation is necessary even with beneficial activities like exercise, because some people could become excessively dependent on exercise, causing both mental and physical health problems.

More reasons the body hungers for physical activity are found in Part 5.

Giving Service

Nothing works as quickly and completely to fill up an aching heart as doing something kind for someone else. Researchers have even reported evidence for why the "do good to feel good" phenomenon works.[49] People who give time, money, or support to others are shown in research to be happier, more satisfied with life, and less depressed.[50]

If you have found yourself emotionally empty and need a boost to get you started, here are three ideas among hundreds out there.

HelpOthers.Org

HelpOthers.Org is a Web site collecting stories about the Smile

---

48. Raglin, J.S (1990) Exercise and mental health, Beneficial and detrimental effects, *Sports Medicine* 9(6): 323-9

49. Moll, J. (2006) Human fronto–mesolimbic networks guide decisions about charitable donation, *Proceedings of the National Academy of Sciences.* 103 (42) 15623-8

50. Farino, L. "Do Good, Feel Good: New research shows that helping others may be the key to happiness" *MSN Health.* Available at http://health.msn.com/health-topics/depression/do-good-feel-good

Card project started by college students. When they noticed that students had lots of energy to do pranks on rival football teams, the students thought of a game to channel some of that energy for a positive purpose. They started a Smile Card challenge in which they did anonymous acts of kindness and left behind a card.

Their project has now mushroomed to over 800,000 Smile Cards distributed in dozens of countries around the world.[51]

SMILE.
You've just been tagged!
**Experiments in Anonymous Kindness
is the name of the game.
And now, YOU'RE IT!**

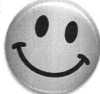

Someone reached out to you with an anonymous act of kindness.
Now it's your chance to do the same.
Do something nice for someone else,
leave this card behind, and keep the spirit going!

Visit **www.helpothers.org** for more ideas, info and inspiration.

The fragrance always remains on the hand that gives the rose. -Gandhi

---

51. http://www.helpothers.org

Kiva

Kiva is a non-profit group that makes micro-credit loans to help bring people out of poverty. They offer a network where individuals can lend as little as $25 at a time to needy individuals through established microfinance institutions in 59 different countries. With the loans, low income people start small businesses to support their families, and they pay the money back with an impressive 98.9% repayment rate.

Started in 2005, there are now over 700,000 lenders who have donated over $316 million. The lenders are individuals from every walk of life who get to read about the progress their $25 helps to fund. Lenders even get the money back at the end of the year, to keep or to relend to someone else.

Read more about the projects and opportunities at the Kiva Web site.[52]

Random Acts of Kindness Foundation

Random Acts of Kindness Foundation is "an internationally recognized non-profit organization founded upon the powerful belief in kindness and dedicated to providing resources and tools that encourage acts of kindness."[53]

Their Web site collects stories about people who use their skills to inspire optimism and change. They sponsor Random Acts of Kindness Week every February and encourage members with resources, curriculum ideas for teachers, and a free newsletter.

All of these service organizations share the amazing conclusion that while trying to do good for others, even greater benefits of

---

52. http://www.kiva.org/lend
53. http://www.randomactsofkindness.org/
54. http://www.helpothers.org/story.php?sid=31133

satisfaction are received by those who perform the service. Their Web sites are full of stories about emotional boosts like this one: [54]

> Last week, in an unusual way, a stranger showered me with generosity.
>
> At an Asian grocery store on a busy evening, I was shopping for the items I needed for my volunteer work of cooking breakfast on Saturday at a homeless shelter in San Jose. I went to the store to buy tofu and fruit. As I was waiting in line to finish the purchase, the lady next to me approached me to find out how I was going to consume the big box of tofu I was buying. Enthusiastically, I replied that I was buying food for the homeless breakfast feed.
>
> While I was getting ready to pay the bill, to my amazement, she offered to pay for everything. Despite multiple requests for her name, she responded that she felt good because I was doing the kind of community work her parents once received when they came to this country as refugees. Hence she wanted to take the opportunity to show her gratitude.
>
> It was the best reward I had ever received for my volunteer work, which began three years ago.
>
> In a strange way we all are connected and feel for each other. That's what I call being a "human."

Work to Understand and Relieve World Hunger

As you address your own emotional hunger, consider those suffering from ongoing poverty and true hunger throughout the world. Helping them can give you great satisfaction and truly fill you up emotionally.

A longer discussion of what world hunger looks like and what you can do about it is provided in Chapters 61 and 62.

Professional Help

Significant unmet emotional needs may require professional help to understand and satisfy. In some cases, counseling (and if necessary, medications) may be needed to treat mental health issues that people have addressed by overeating.

FingerTIPS about Emotional Emptiness

- Look for "hunger" messages in poetry, literature, and scriptures, and start noticing your own hunger-related emotions.

- Test your physical hunger by concentrating on the center of your abdomen, and use the 5-point scale to give yourself a satiety rating (see Chapter 18). When you are familiar with your body's *satiety* signals you can be more aware of emotional needs.

- Track your hunger ratings, including both physical and emotional cues to eat, over three days or one week.

- Assess your stress level and read about stress management techniques.

- Modify recipes for your favorite comfort foods so they are healthier, reduce guilt, and fill you up physically with fewer calories. See sample recipe at the end of this section.

- Experiment with new ways to fill your emotional emptiness such as intellectual stimulation, physical activity, or giving service and working on world hunger.

Emotional Fullness Quiz

IF YOU WERE to experience the following, estimate your likely reaction with one of these ratings:

5 = strong desire to eat

4 = mild desire to eat

3 = no effect on eating

2 = no desire to eat

1 = strong aversion to eating

_____ A. Your favorite candidate lost the election.

_____ B. You are tired of being in school and wish you were done.

_____ C. You are living a long distance from home and wish you were there.

_____ D. You are worried about the results of a biopsy you had.

_____ E. You are nervous about a presentation you have to make at work in front of top management.

_____ F. You just got news that you were turned down for the job you interviewed for, which you really wanted.

_____ G. Your friend is in pain and you feel inadequate to do anything to help.

_____ H. Your pet died after a long illness.

_____ I. You just got news that you won a scholarship.

_____ J. You are worried that you might not be able to afford the home you want to buy.

Add up your scores.

Emotional Quiz Scoring

If you scored lower than 30, the third hunger of emotional emptiness is not your primary hunger.

If you scored higher than 30,

- Identify the foods you would usually turn to as comfort foods.

- If your favorite foods are not the healthiest ones for your current needs, see the Comfort Food Makeover.

- Feed your emptiness as described in Chapter 34 with intellectual stimulation, physical activity, or giving service and working on world hunger.

36

Resources about Emotional Eating

FOLLOWING ARE SOME helpful books and articles to explore for more information as you become more aware of the third hunger.

Mayo Clinic, (2009), *"Weight Loss Help: Gain Control of Emotional Eating,"* available at http://www.mayoclinic.com/health/weight-loss/MH00025

Explains how emotional eating can sabotage your weight-loss efforts and provides tips to regain control of your eating habits.

Van Hart, Zach, *"Get a Handle on Emotional Eating: The Secret Sabotage of Your Program"* by *SparkPeople* ®, available at http://www.sparkpeople.com

Harding, Ann, (2011), *"Study Offers Clues to Emotional Eating,"* CNN Health, available at http://www.cnn.com/2011/HEALTH/07/25/study.clues.emotional.eating/index.html

Psychology Today, *Emotional Eating Test.*

Interactive test with 149 questions, partial results free, full results with personalized interpretation, available for purchase at http://psychologytoday.tests.psychtests.com/take_test.php?idRegTest=1599

Hatfield, Heather, (2003), *"Emotional Eating: Feeding Your Feelings,"* Eating to feed a feeling, and not a growling stomach, is emotional eating, *WebMD Feature*, available at http://www.webmd.com/diet/features/emotional-eating-feeding-your-feelings

Tribole, Evelyn & Resch Elyse, (2003), *Intuitive Eating: A Revolutionary Program That Works,* St Martin's Press

Focuses on nurturing your body rather than starving it, encourages natural weight loss, and helps you find the weight you were meant to be.

37

FingerFOODS
Recipe for the Third Hunger

ONCE YOU RECOGNIZE when your hunger is in response to one of your many emotional needs, you can make a decision to feed the true hunger.

In the meantime, try a traditional comfort food made over to be a healthy addition to your meals. The healthier version will leave you feeling more full and less guilty!

Makeover Mashed Potatoes

Try a variety of vegetables, steamed and mashed, to replace or add to traditional mashed potatoes.

The following work well in mashed and creamy form:
- Cauliflower
- Parsnips
- Butternut Squash
- Pumpkin

Peel and slice vegetables into 1-inch slices.

Bring to boil and simmer on low heat until tender, about 12 minutes. Drain, retaining liquid.

Mash in food processor or by hand. Add back some of the liquid to desired consistency. Lightly salt to taste.

TIP: Mash an orange vegetable (cooked carrot or squash) in with white vegetables (cauliflower, potatoes or parsnips) for a buttery appearance that will fool your taste buds while being fat free!

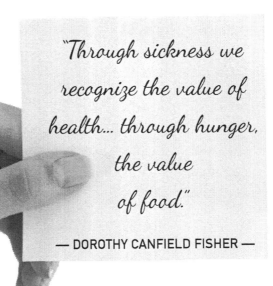

"Through sickness we recognize the value of health... through hunger, the value of food."

— DOROTHY CANFIELD FISHER —

PART IV

The Ring Finger

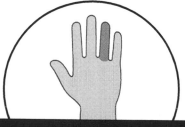

The Fourth Hunger Is for Stability

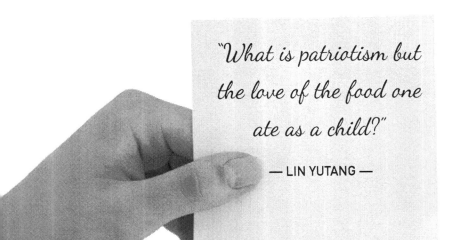

"What is patriotism but
the love of the food one
ate as a child?"

— LIN YUTANG —

38

The Parable of Navajo Frybread

MAYBE YOU ARE familiar with Navajo frybread, the puffy fried pancake common in the southwest U.S. People often eat it with various toppings such as honey or as a Navajo Taco, made by adding lettuce, tomatoes, beans, and cheese. The tasty treats are staples at county fairs. Frybread is ubiquitous among some Native American tribes, eaten daily and celebrated at powwows.

However, in 2005 the USDA listed frybread as a high fat food, showing that a slice the size of a large paper plate could contain 700 calories and 25 grams of fat.[55] To put that in perspective, an average glazed donut contains about 250 calories and 12 grams of fat.

The USDA warned that these high fat foods led to increased health risks. Native Americans were outraged. How could the USDA attack one of their favorite foods? More importantly, frybread is a cultural symbol. They had been eating frybread for generations. The name "Navajo Frybread" conferred a unique status. How many other foods are widely recognized as "Navajo" in origin?

To add insult to injury, one of their own agreed with the USDA.

Editor and activist Suzan Shown Harjo wrote a column in the newsletter *Indian Country Today* [56] that challenged the traditional

---

55. USDA, available at http://ndb.nal.usda.gov/ndb/foods/show/7534

56. Miller, J. (2008) Frybead: This seemingly simple food is a complicated symbol in Navajo culture, *Smithsonian Magazine* July, 2008, available at http://www.smithsonianmag.com/people-places/frybread.html#ixzz1vTPPViTM

notion that frybread was a legitimate cultural icon. "Frybread is emblematic of the long trails from home and freedom to confinement and rations. It's the connecting dot between healthy children and obesity, hypertension, diabetes, dialysis, blindness, amputations, and slow death. If frybread were a movie, it would be hard-core porn. No redeeming qualities. Zero nutrition."

Harjo researched the origin of this popular meal. Navajo frybread was invented in 1863 at a tragic point in Native American history. When the U.S. Army forced Indians off their land, in illegal defiance of existing treaties, the beleaguered and starving indigenous people were given rations of flour, salt, and lard as they followed the 300-mile "Long Walk" to New Mexico. They had to abandon their true cultural foods of elk, buffalo, corn, beans, and squash.

These Native Americans showed remarkable ingenuity and resourcefulness, using the Army rations to make a portable high-calorie trail food to support them on their march, and frybread was born. Both during the strenuous Long Walk and in their new home in the New Mexico desert, their rigorous lifestyles required high calories—and frybread supplied them. They kept eating it as new generations were born, and it became a favorite food.

But now, flash forward to the 21st century where the Indian people are as *sedentary* (physically inactive) as the rest of the U.S., and the frybread supplies many more calories than they need. What they considered part of their cultural heritage is now killing them. They suffer from diabetes and other obesity-related diseases at rates higher than any other population group. The overall prevalence of diabetes in 2002 was two to three times higher for American Indian adults than for U.S. adults.[57]

Native American musician Keith Secola said, "Frybread has killed more Indians than the federal government." Secola wrote a

---

57. CDC (2003) *MMWR Weekly* August 1, 2003 / 52(30);702-704, available at http://www.cdc.gov/mmwr/preview/mmwrhtml/mm5230a3.htm

song called *Frybread*, celebrating the favorite food and calling it a cultural symbol of both perseverance and pain. He also laments that frybread is a scapegoat for the lack of healthful food, nutritional education, and good access to health care.

I call the story of Navajo frybread a parable. Although it is a true story for Native Americans, it is also an allegory for what American food has done to the population as a whole.

A similar theme was reported by Morgan Spurlock in the documentary he produced, *Super Size Me*.[58] To make his film, he experimented on himself by eating three meals per day at McDonalds, for thirty days. He included a commentary on the fast food habits of Americans and the mushrooming health problems from our collective overconsumption.

In 2004 when his film won the Grand Jury Prize at the Sundance Film Festival, I attended the public screening where Spurlock responded to audience questions after the film. One of his comments was reminiscent of how the Native Americans defended frybread. Spurlock said that during the making of his movie when he interviewed people across the country, they were defensive when he criticized America's favorite foods. People felt that burgers and fries were all-American and a cultural icon.

As Spurlock's film pointed out, burgers and fries are not vintage American foods handed down from our ancestral heritage. (Hamburgers are not even American in origin, as their name stems from Hamburg, Germany. Hot dogs, or frankfurters, are from Frankfurt, Germany.) Popular fast foods such as tacos and pizza barely resemble the healthy foods in their nations of origin. When is the last time you had beans and rice in a tortilla and called it a taco? You've probably had meat and cheese, at a minimum.

I still remember the first time I had a taco. Back in the 1960s

---

58. Spurlock, M. (2004) *Super Size Me*, Morgan Spurlock Projects, available at http://morganspurlock.com/super-size-me/

we were living in Wisconsin, and my sister came home from college. She'd discovered all sorts of new foods in the exotic food capital of Provo, Utah.

One of them was tacos.

My sister made us a fun new meal she had learned from her college roommate. We were amazed at the unusual concoction! It was the first taco we had ever seen—a corn tortilla holding a little ground beef and grated cheese, covered by lettuce and tomatoes. Of course this was more than forty years ago.

Now you can get a taco loaded up with the works—at Taco Bell it's called a DOUBLE DECKER Taco Supreme—at any time of the day. It provides 350 calories, with 140 from fat. It only has 3 grams of sugar, but the 670 mg of sodium is more than 1/3 of the daily amount recommended by the American Heart Association.

Or, you could have Volcano Nachos, with 990 calories (550 from fat), with 1570 mg of sodium and 6 g of sugar. Get that with a 40 oz Mountain Dew and add 550 calories, 150 mg of sodium, and 145 g of sugar.

Don't even get me started on pizza!

So am I advocating that we boycott fast foods and avoid frybread?

No! The message here is simply to start learning more about where your food preferences have really come from—and to discard the illusion that unhealthy foods are our inevitable favorites.

The food industry spends millions of dollars to form people's food preferences. They are remarkably successful too. It's no wonder so much advertising is targeted at young children. Once we have ingrained preferences, we accept these new habits as necessities and cling to them without questioning.

Which brings us to the fourth hunger: the hunger for stability. Much of our eating is just out of habit, because we love the stability of eating the same things we have been eating for months and years.

✦ 39 ✦

The Need for Stability

WE WERE IN Mumbai, India, on a Sunday and wanted to visit one of our church buildings for Sunday services. We found a cab driver who agreed to take us. The building was in Navi Mumbai, a suburb across the river that he said he was familiar with. We had printed out the directions, including a sheet that showed the exact route with a blue line on the map, but our driver only wanted the address. He was uninterested in the map.

When we had passed the turnoff, we told the driver. He pulled over. We showed him the map, where we were, and how to get back to where we wanted to go. The driver looked at it for a minute and then waved down a family that was standing at the side of the road. Speaking Hindi, he asked the man how to get to the address. The man responded with a long explanation, and the cab driver drove exactly the way our map showed.

Until we came to the cross streets.

Again we tried to show him the map. He looked at it again, but instead asked three more pedestrians how to get to the address.

Eventually we reached our destination, but it was amusing to see the driver persist in his habit of asking for directions instead of consulting a map. We thought it was likely he'd never used maps; certainly he didn't have one in his car. (And he didn't have a GPS, either.)

The need for stability is the fourth stealth appetite. It's usually manifested by our habits. This may be the stealthiest of the appetites because we don't even realize it is an appetite!

Like our unnecessarily wayward driving adventure in Mumbai, our lives tend toward chaos. We're hit constantly with unexpected health problems, financial reverses, and interpersonal conflicts. Apart from the inevitability of aging, there's no set pattern in the way our lives unfold. Consequently, we have a hunger for stability and balance. This hunger is so strong that we develop patterns—habits—that remove at least some of the uncertainty and chaos.

Like the Russian dolls that contain ever smaller dolls within, we have habits within habits within habits. Millions of Americans come home at night (habit) and watch TV (habit). And what's TV if not a predictable pattern? Shows are 30 or 60 minutes long. Each show starts with a conflict. The resolution of that conflict leads to a greater conflict, and so on in a three-act structure first described by Aristotle thousands of years ago. By the end of the designated period, the conflicts are resolved, and we're satisfied. Unlike in our real lives, the fiction we watch has a fulfilling completion—a beginning, middle, and end. This pattern is so consistent that an experienced movie critic can tell you exactly when the plot twists will occur, even in a movie he has never seen before.

Because they help us make sense of the world—without them life is too chaotic—our habits are deeply ingrained. They are subconscious, embedded in our natures like our heartbeats are embedded in our bodies. We don't consciously command our hearts to beat; likewise, we don't consciously think about our habits.

But we can.

And we must, if those habits contradict our goals.

The great thing about habits is they can push us forward just as easily as they can hinder us. We're happy our hearts have a "habit" of beating regularly. As we adopt better food and eating habits, we can satisfy the stealth appetite for stability in a productive way.

And if we make goals and write them down, we can consult them like a map. Unlike our cab driver in Mumbai, we won't be constantly asking for directions every time we're lost. We won't get lost in the first place!

Our Bodies Love Habits

OUR LIVES ARE dominated by the habits we have developed through a lifetime of repeating the same behaviors over and over again. Good habits help us each day. We don't have to think about how to take a shower, get dressed, or drive to work. These repeated actions, which have become habits, allow us to now do them without thinking, freeing up brainpower to focus on other things.

Biologically, our organs thrive with the stability of routines such as the circadian rhythms of getting sleepy the same time every evening and springing awake about the same time every morning.

Our intestines process food and eliminate best when on a predictable schedule. (Note that laxatives promise to restore *regularity*.) As reviewed in Part 1, our blood sugar is best in control when the stomach, pancreas, and other organs receive food to process at predictable times each day.

Our behavior also responds in a similar way to predictable routines that become ingrained habits. When we have repeated an action to the point that it has created synaptic pathways in our brain, eventually we stop thinking about the original reason behind the action, and it simply becomes a habit.

Once we have deeply-rooted food preferences, both our minds and bodies expect those same foods on a routine basis, and we start perceiving them not just as preferences but as needs.

The challenge of the fourth hunger is to determine, whenever we want to eat, whether we are truly physically hungry or have simply developed a habit that our body and mind insist we must satisfy or act upon.

Habits Are Stronger than Goals

Changing our eating habits can be one of the most challenging goals we will ever set. Despite our good intentions, the majority of the time a habit we have had for a long time will always be stronger than a goal recently decided. This accounts for the common relapse or recidivism within a few weeks after making New Year's resolutions. Regardless of our desire for a healthier way of eating, our bodies and minds will fight to retain our deeply-ingrained habits. Research has shown that even animals find habits more compelling than enticing new incentives.

While goals take thought, commitment, and a plan to achieve, a habit is automatic. Without conscious thought we will naturally be led in the direction of the habit.

⊹ 41 ⊹

Why Do You Like That Food?

Our food preferences were most likely developed years ago in our infancy. Likes and dislikes were formed based on habits and availability. For example, Mom fed us what was available and what she ate growing up. We then developed the habit of eating what was placed before us. These habits then became part of our normal routine.

Even now we probably find ourselves eating the same things our mother fed us, adopting a few of our spouse's eating habits—and teaching them to our children. These habits we picked up are not necessarily bad or good, but they may not be helping us. We need to evaluate our current situations and decide if those eating habits are serving us well or not at this stage in our lives.

If we grew up drinking whole milk, eating white bread and drinking soda, or avoiding fruits and vegetables, then it may be time to change a few of our habits.

One of the community classes I taught over the years was to inmates in the county jail. They were always polite and orderly, but a little surprised by what I told them about the need for healthier food habits. They seemed to doubt that anyone could take nutrition seriously. I would often ask them to name their favorite foods, and answers were predictable, things like pizza or burgers and fries. Then I would pose the question "Why do you like that food?" or "Why is it your favorite?"

I would always get answers like these:

- It's obvious, I want to eat only what I like.

- Everyone knows junk food tastes better.

- If food is healthy, it does not taste good.

- If it tastes good, it must be bad for you.

- I refuse to eat what the food police want to make me eat.

Students in my college classes write in their beginning essays that we need to *"eat healthier."* But when I press them about what that means, most of them draw a blank. Those who offer some specifics usually spout clichés that are often untrue. Their ideas of healthy eating include cutting out carbs, eating unlimited protein, eating unlimited fat (as long as it is not trans fat), or always choosing chicken or salad over anything else. Basically, they are getting their information from what the media has said is good. Unfortunately, that is often inaccurate and almost always confusing.

Peer pressure can play a big part in determining our preferences, and researchers have found evidence of it in children as young as age four. Take this scenario, for example.

Four-year-old Sammy is in preschool. The teacher asks Sammy what he would like for a snack and he answers, "Carrots!" So, Sammy's teacher gives him a small bag of carrots and he starts to eat them happily. A few minutes later Bobby comes up and sees the bag of carrots. With a disgusted look, he says, "Carrots are yucky!" Sammy slowly puts down the carrot. Later, when the teacher comes back, she says "Hey Sammy, why didn't you finish your carrots?" Sammy looks at the carrots with a disgusted look on his face and answers, "I don't like carrots, carrots are yucky!"

Adult Peer Pressure: The Media

Children are not the only ones affected by peer pressure. As adults we are influenced both by our friends and by the "imaginary friends" we see on TV and in movies.

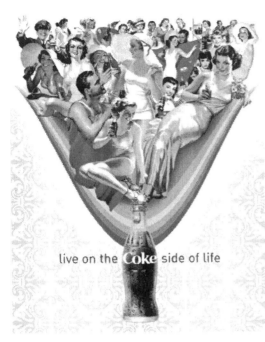

live on the Coke side of life

This vintage ad shows that CocaCola was marketed by providing people some imaginary peers and leading them to believe they must like Coke if all these happy and beautiful people do.

Burger King had a famous ad campaign in the 1970s where they targeted specific population groups to convince them that people just like their families loved Whoppers and fries.

Remember, the food industry spends millions to form people's food preferences—and they are remarkably successful at it.

Chapulines

Here's a tasty snack you might like—have you ever eaten *chapulines?* They are a favorite food in Oaxaca, Mexico. You will find tables piled with chapulines at roadside vendors, and they are served in many Mexican restaurants in the U.S. They are crunchy and well-seasoned with garlic, lime, or chiles. Sound good?

Chapulines are roasted grasshoppers! They are thoroughly cleaned, then toasted and seasoned. They are high in protein, B vitamins, iron and zinc, and they're low in fat. Great nutrition!

Chapulines may not be your favorite food, but the choices we make, based on what our culture has taught is "normal," may seem equally unappetizing to others. If you had grown up in Oaxaca, you would probably love chapulines, but you might hate some foods typical in the U.S.

I know several people who have moved to the U.S. from Oaxaca. So far, every one of them has told me they hate Root Beer. They cringe when it is offered and say they cannot imagine how anyone would drink it, let alone enjoy it. When they ask me why I like it, I tell them the same reason we all like certain foods—because I learned to like it from early childhood.

— 42 —

Food Preferences Can Be Changed!

OF ALL THE REASONS someone may think about changing their food choices, health issues are the most common. Consider two cases from my experience as a hospital dietitian. Most people fall into two categories, like Mr. A and Mr. B.

Their doctor told both men that their blood pressure was high, and they would need to start a low sodium diet. They were dismayed. They both said they would never be able to adjust to unsalted food and were sure the food would taste terrible, ensuring they would never be able to enjoy food again. I challenged them both to try it for one week and tell me how it went.

Mr. A reported later that he could not stand the unsalted hospital food and had someone smuggle in food from outside the hospital. Sure enough, at the end of the week, unsalted food still tasted unpleasant to him.

Mr. B. reported that at first he could not eat the food. However, the second day he was hungry enough to try some, and choked it down. The third day he tried it again, and the fourth day he felt he was starting to get used to it. By the fifth and sixth day he noticed new flavors and realized they were better than the former salty taste. By the end of the week he said he preferred this new way of eating and requested that we give him only unsalted food in the future.

The difference here was in the attitudes of the men. Because Mr. B was willing to give it a try, was open to a change, and stayed with the change despite the discomfort of challenging a long-standing habit, he achieved a different result.

Like Mr. A and Mr. B, most Americans would profit by cutting down on excess sodium in their foods, since we eat almost twice the recommended limit daily. Unfortunately, even eliminating the salt shaker will not be enough to keep our meals at a healthy sodium level, because salt we add at the table accounts for only 11% of the sodium we eat.[59] Nearly 80% is added to foods in the processing. This is another reason to reject processed foods that advertisers tell us we like, and rely more on fruits and vegetables!

Like saltiness, sweetness is an acquired taste and a habit that can be a challenge to change. But many people, after cutting sugar out of their diet, state that they notice the sweetness of foods more than they did before. In addition, many have trouble going back to eating sweet foods and would have to adjust their preferences again to incorporate sweet food into their daily diet.

Food Addiction?

Some researchers have suggested that food addictions, a controversial concept, are similar to substance abuse. High fat and high sugar foods stimulate the brain using the same pathways used by addictive drugs.

Excessive intake of sugars and fats may or may not indicate a true addiction. Nevertheless, it is helpful to know that when you feel somehow "dependent" on sweets or your preferred comfort foods, it is not your imagination but a deeply-ingrained habit that both your body and brain have grown to expect.

As with drugs, people can develop a tolerance to certain foods, needing more of them to feel satisfied. Like drug addicts, they may

---

59. New York City Department of Health and Mental Hygiene, "Cutting Salt, Improving Health," available at http://www.nyc.gov/html/doh/html/cardio/cardio-salt-initiative.shtml

continue to eat large quantities of unhealthy foods in spite of negative consequences. Similar to addictions, suddenly removing a food they have come to depend on may cause symptoms of withdrawal.

Despite the strength of food preferences and habits, they *can* be changed. You can even harness the habit-forming properties of foods to make your habits work in your behalf instead of against you.

43

The Struggle to Change a Habit

ON ONE FATEFUL winter day last year, I slipped on the ice and badly fractured my kneecap. The mishap came at a bad time, as we were scheduled to leave that day on a cross-country flight to attend a wedding. Luckily I was able to splint up my leg and get onboard anyway, a few hours after my fall (although I don't recommend that if you can help it).

I was fortunate to receive competent medical care. After surgery to wire the kneecap back together and six weeks of keeping my leg straight, the bone healed successfully.

Then began the slow process of physical therapy working to train my knee to bend again and strengthen the weakened muscles. I was amazed at what a strong new *habit* my leg had acquired. My leg now was most comfortable straight and it refused to bend. It was difficult and painful even to bend it slightly.

My goal was clear—I wanted to walk with a normal healthy gait, but my leg's new habit made that temporarily impossible.

Several times each day I wanted to revert to my comfortable old habit, to sit in the recliner with my leg up. But when I remembered my goal to walk normally again, it was enough incentive to work through the discomfort to change the straight leg habit and re-learn to bend my knee. I had not realized it would take more than six months to feel comfortable walking again. The whole ordeal taught me lessons that are also true in changing habits for healthier eating.

44

Habit Lessons Learned

THE FIRST POINT was one that many of my students and clients have difficulty accepting. My broken bone and surgery were not a choice but the result of external forces. Due to circumstances out of my control, I ended up with a serious obstacle—a stiff knee.

The ruts we get in (eating high-fat and high-sugar foods) are not a conscious choice to be unhealthy but a result of external factors, including our hectic schedules, our food culture, the influence of advertising, peer pressure, and the food scientists that make these foods so irresistible. Once we accept the reality of our situation and the obstacles we face, we're ready to deal with them.

When I discovered the bone was healed but my knee would no longer bend, I had to choose. I could either be comfortable but deal with a stiff leg the rest of my life, or go through the difficult process of re-training my leg to walk normally.

When we evaluate our health and realize we have developed unhealthy habits, we can choose to stay that way and limp through life with poor health and low energy, or make the challenging changes to re-train our eating and activity patterns. We don't have to accept the circumstances into which life has placed us.

I frequently wanted to take a short cut; I thought if I worked hard in a burst, I could push the knee to speed up the process. Two or three times I worked so hard I developed tendonitis or other strains leading to setbacks in the process. My physical therapist had to remind me often, "Slow is fast!"

It is normal to want a crash diet or fast change to immediately make everything different. Drastic sudden changes in eating habits often create other problems, which usually include giving up. We have to constantly remind ourselves, *slow is fast*. Because we want the changes to last, we must patiently and gradually work at them until they feel natural.

I had to deal with emotional challenges. Having my mobility impaired was demoralizing. I did not want to admit that I could not walk fast, walk upstairs, or hike in the mountains (let alone run). I couldn't even drive a car. I thought I was a wimp if I had to stop and rest or admit my leg was too sore for more exercise. It helped greatly that family and friends reassured me and gave moral support (as well as rides wherever I needed to go, although sitting in the back seat with my leg stretched out wasn't so much fun).

When we develop unhealthy habits we have to be kind to ourselves and not beat ourselves up. These are habits, not moral failings. We can patiently change them and plan optimistically for the day when our overall health will be improved. Meanwhile we have to remember to reward ourselves with fun and healthy alternatives. We need to surround ourselves with supportive friends and family. We need kindness from others and from ourselves.

45

Make Habits Work <u>FOR</u> You

SINCE OUR HABITS are stronger than our goals, and most people go through life blindly led by their habits, it may seem we are hopeless victims of our past and change is impossible. That has been the attitude of hundreds of my weight-loss clients. But they overlook an important truth—the same principle works for good habits!

Once we establish healthy habits that are aligned with our goals and we set consciously-decided patterns, healthier eating and activity will be incorporated systematically in our routines. At that point our goals will have become our unconscious habits.

Habit Change Research

Martin Grunburg, author of *The Habit Factor*,[60] has built a successful business on the premise that habit is what drives goal achievement. His book gives specific guidance on habit change to reach your goals and replacing bad habits with good habits.

Dan & Chip Heath wrote a popular book on changing habits called *Switch*,[61] and used the example of trying to change eating habits as one of the most difficult endeavors humans undertake.

60. Grunburg, M., (2010) *The Habit Factor®: An Innovative Method to Align Habits with Goals to Achieve Success*, Equilibrium Enterprises, La Jolla, CA

61. Heath, C. and Heath D., (2010) *Switch: How to Change Things When Change Is Hard*. Broadway Books, New York

They suggested that the three essential elements in all change are (1) mental clarity, (2) emotional motivation, and (3) situational preparedness. It is easy to see why food habits are difficult to change—all three of those elements are especially challenging when it comes to our food preferences and food habits.

Mental clarity

Nutrition is controversial and emotional, and there are hundreds of disagreements among both consumers and nutritionists about what is healthiest to eat. Some advocates are motivated by commercial interests—they have a product to sell. Others are motivated by scientific findings, but even these sometimes reflect a particular agenda.

Before making a change in eating habits a person should understand his or her body's needs and what foods will fill those needs. Simpler is better, which is why I suggest working on a few basic changes before trying for a dramatic overhaul.

Emotional Motivation

The emotional side is what most often undermines success in habit change. This is important to note—if you cannot change a habit, it is not due to a failure of will power—instead it is the triumph of your body's struggle to maintain stability.

As discussed in Part 3, emotional reasons for eating often overshadow our body's physical needs. Making any change will upset the careful balance our habits have set in place and will require enormous support. Change is possible, but not trivial.

I recommend reinforcing any habit change with large doses of emotional support from others. Enlist the support of family and friends. And use resources such as detailed in Part 3—intellectual stimulation, physical activity and giving service.

Situational Preparedness: Environmental Factors

Before making any change in your habits, consider your environment and anticipate the ambient forces that will either support or undermine your efforts. Some ideas to get you started are included in the next chapter.

✦ 46 ✦

Your Food Environment

BEFORE YOU ARE ready to make a change in your eating habits, you will need to study and address the environment in which you live, work, and eat. Think about what we learned about the supermarket pharmacy. Then look at the following two photos and ask yourself which is more representative of your surroundings?

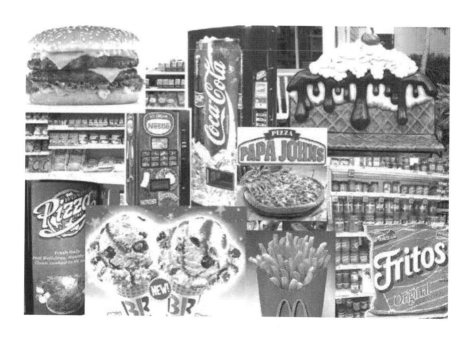

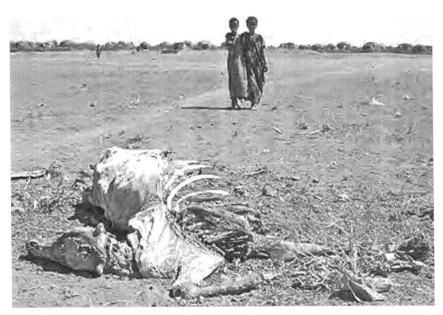

The first photo is part of our everyday lives, and it seems normal until viewed in contrast to the second one. Seeing them together is a dramatic display of what has been called our *toxic food environment*.

Consider how advertising and the media can saturate our lives with foods. While we once thought of a cookie as an occasional treat, the collective consciousness now considers constant desserts and snacks as normal.

Just as smokers trying to quit will distance themselves from reminders of tobacco, you can make a healthy habit change much easier if you create a healthy food environment for yourself.

Take the following *Food Environment Assessment* as you consider your own surroundings. You will probably need to take the list with you for observation during the day, as most people are only vaguely aware of these until they consciously go looking for them.

Food Environment Assessment

1. How many open candy dishes are on counters, tables, or desks at home and in your office?

2. How many food photos are on billboards on your most commonly traveled routes? What foods are in the photos?

3. How many food and beverage vending machines do you walk by in your normal routine?

4. How many commercials for food come on during the hours you most often watch TV? What is being advertised?

5. How many fast-food restaurants do you drive by on your most commonly-traveled routes?

6. How many colorful food photos are on the cover or near the front of your favorite magazines? What foods are in the photos?

And, most uncomfortable for some people, right in your own home:

7. What foods are visible as you walk through your house?

8. In what room(s) is food readily available?

9. Which foods are most accessible in your kitchen and require little preparation?

10. When you open your refrigerator, which foods do you see first?

11. Has food storage overflowed into hallways or counters because you don't have enough cupboards or storage closets?

Create your own healthier food environment by first being conscious of what surrounds you. Then make changes to reinforce your own healthy preferences. Some basic principles are:

- Enlist the help of your household's food gatekeeper (especially if it is yourself) to keep healthier foods on hand and to stop supplying foods you want to avoid.

- Put food away: out of sight is out of mind.

- Don't buy more food than you have room to store.

- Hang pictures of your favorite calming scenery instead of favorite foods

- Be aware of food photos on magazine covers, and turn them over or store on a shelf.

- Organize your refrigerator and food pantry with your healthiest foods most accessible.

- Be aware of food cues and influences in your school or work setting, and change your routes if needed to avoid constant food reminders.

FingerTIPS about the Hunger for Stability

- Our bodies love habits and crave stability in routines, foods, activity patterns, and our surroundings.

- Food preferences originate early in life and can be heavily influenced by peers, advertising, and the media.

- Our habits become so ingrained they may feel like necessities.

- Habits are stronger than goals and often undermine our success in trying to eat healthier.

- High sugar and high fat foods create especially strong habits that are much like addictions.

- Food preferences and habits *can* be changed, but the efforts to create healthy habits require significant attention.

- Use helpful resources from habit change research to assess and change your eating patterns.

- Consider your emotional needs and enlist help to support the transition, as your changes will inevitably upset your body's craving for stability.

- Structure your personal environment to reinforce the changes you want to make.

✛ 48 ✛
Resources about Habit Change

Aldana, Steven, (2005), *The Culprit and the Cure: Why Lifestyle Is the Culprit Behind America's Poor Health,* Maple Mountain Press

> Explains in a light-hearted but scientifically supported way how the average person can make effective lifestyle changes in diet and exercise.

Claiborn, James & Pedrick, Cherry, (2001), *The Habit Change Workbook: How to Break Bad Habits and Form Good Ones,* New Harbinger Publications, Oakland, CA

> This step-by-step, cognitive-behavioral program helps you break unwanted habits and replace them with healthy new ones. This book has been awarded The Association for Behavioral and Cognitive Therapies Self-Help Seal of Merit.

Duhigg, Charles, (2012), *The Power of Habit: Why We Do What We Do in Life and Business,* Random House, New York.

> Combines research and stories about how habits shape our lives and how we can shape our habits.

Heath, Chip & Heath, Dan, (2010), *Switch: How to Change Things When Change Is Hard,* Broadway Books, New York

> The Heaths bring together research in psychology, sociology,

and other fields about how we can effect transformative change. *Switch* shows that successful changes follow a pattern you can use in changing the world or changing your waistline.

Ryan, M.J., (2006), *This Year I Will . . . . How to Finally Change a Habit, Keep a Resolution, or Make a Dream Come True,* Broadway Books, New York

Learn the secret to making changes that stick. Breakthrough wisdom and coaching to help readers make *this time* the time that change becomes permanent.

Selig, Meg, (2009), *Changepower!: 37 Secrets to Habit Change Success,* Taylor & Francis, New York

A step-by-step process to achieve any habit change goal. First-person stories, pithy quotes, and how-to exercises provide inspiration, humor, and encouragement as readers embark on their habit change journeys.

✦ 49 ✦
FingerFOODS
Recipe for the Fourth Hunger

MOST OF US tend to limit ourselves to the foods we have known and loved for years. One way to introduce yourself and your family to healthy new foods is to disguise them as old favorites.

Break a habit and learn to love tofu while you think you're eating good old scrambled eggs. Tofu is worth introducing—low in calories, lactose-free, very high in complete protein, but free of cholesterol and saturated fats.

Tofu Scramble (you'll swear it's eggs)

1 14- to 16-oz block of firm tofu
½ cup chopped green onions
1 clove garlic, crushed (optional)
1 Tbsp olive oil
Salt and pepper

Sauté onion and garlic in oil. Drain tofu and mash with fork into sautéed vegetables, heat 5 minutes. Salt and pepper to taste. Best if served while warm. Note: tofu will not overcook (as eggs will) if kept warm.

Optional toppings:
- Bacon or substitute
- Diced fresh tomatoes
- Grated cheese
- Your favorite omelet fillings

Makes 4 servings, each the size of two eggs.

"Hunger is not only the best cook, but also the best physician."

— PORTUGUESE PROVERB —

PART V

The Pinky

The Fifth Hunger Is for Novelty

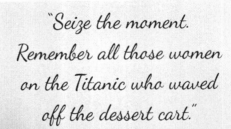

"Seize the moment. Remember all those women on the Titanic who waved off the dessert cart."

— ERMA BOMBECK —

The Fun Hunger

As we've made our way across the fingers of our hands, we've seen how human biology and psychology compel us toward certain behaviors. It's not "fun" to hunger for sugar; it's just something we feel compelled to do. The reward might be considered fun, but the consequences are definitely not. The other three hungers carry a sense of obligation. Physical hunger motivates eating to supply the body's needs. Emotional hunger prompts us to respond to emotional gaps or emptiness. Habits are similar to the automatic functions of our heartbeat and breathing.

But there's also an element of human nature that craves variety and just plain old fun.

I like to think of the fifth finger—the pinky—as the slightly crazy one. Even the name is a little fanciful. "Pinky." Kind of makes you smile, doesn't it?

Even on a keyboard, the right pinky finger handles punctuation, not letters (except for its own—the letter "P"). The left pinky handles Q and A and Z, the oddest combination assigned to any finger.

So when we think of the pinky, we ought to think of doing things differently. Variety. Change. Vacation. Recess. Or just plain fun.

Consider the difference between Adeline and Zak:

Adeline lived in 1862. Her daily routine included hauling wood to replenish the stove before breakfast, feeding the chickens, milking the cows, weeding her vegetable garden, and kneading the dough to make bread. She occasionally walked two miles to the general store for provisions and sometimes treated herself to a piece of molasses candy. For recreation she attended square dances where her favorite was the Virginia Reel.

Zak, on the other hand, is a product of our current modern lifestyle. His daily routine includes walking to the kitchen where his meals are ready for him in the refrigerator, driving to work, and watching TV in the evening. When he needs clothes or supplies he orders them online. Every evening he feels restless and treats himself to ice cream and cookies. For recreation, he watches a movie or plays a video game.

Adeline never once went to a gym to workout, or did calisthenics, or ran a mile on the track. She was probably unaware of her body's need for exercise. Hard physical labor was simply a part of her everyday routine, and she was constantly involved with physical activity.

Zak however is significantly deficient in physical activity but does not realize it. He does feel a vague discomfort every evening as he sits in his recliner and turns on the 6 o'clock news. What he does not recognize is that his body is craving movement. He has been sitting all day—in the car, at his desk and during meals. He sits to socialize with friends on his computer and to play his video games. His body is tired of sitting! He is craving a change in something but is not sure what.

Unfortunately, many of us (like Zak) do not notice the subtle cues that we need to move around. Although our organ systems love the stability of a set routine (as described in Part 4), our skeleton, joints, and circulatory systems were put together to optimize moving around rather than sitting still. Long stretches of inactivity create problems and discomfort.

Also unfortunate is how Zak and many of us respond to the discomfort. We sense the hunger for a change but instead of getting up to stretch or walk around the block or ride a bike, we give ourselves novelty in the form of snacks and sweets.

This is a paradox and the greatest challenge of the fifth hunger—when the change we need most is some physical exercise, we often take a shortcut of calming the restlessness by eating. Food is immediately rewarding and serves to temporarily distract us from the real source of the restlessness, but our bodies never receive the movement break they need.

The same is true of how we react to boredom. The novelty we crave can be temporarily fed with food and drink—our taste buds welcome new sensory experiences. But the food solution is short-lived, causes unwanted side effects, and demands repeating, which shows that it is not the kind of novelty we really hunger for.

A Sedentary Epidemic

The conveniences of modern life have created a new health problem that our ancestors did not dream of—a sedentary lifestyle.

Sedentary means physically inactive and describes Americans in higher numbers than ever before. One recent study by Dr. Frank Hu of the Harvard School of Public Health identified TV viewing as the most prevalent sedentary behavior in our culture.[62] His study reaffirmed what we all know, that inactivity adds to health risks for diabetes, heart disease, and early death. However, this study went further to identify how much TV we watch and predict just how much it increases the risk.

Europeans and Australians spend up to four hours a day watching TV, but Americans top the charts, averaging five hours of TV watching every day. According to the relative risk Dr. Hu

---

62. Grontved, A. & Hu, F. "Television Viewing and Risk of Type 2 Diabetes, Cardiovascular Disease, and All-Cause Mortality: A Meta-analysis" *Journal of the American Medical Association* 305(23):2448-2455

calculated, this would mean 780,000 premature deaths per year of Americans due to excessive television watching. The TV is not directly killing people of course, but being sedentary while watching is preventing Americans from participating in the activity their bodies are hungering for.

Too Much Rest = Fatigue

Everyone needs to rest, but in a lifestyle that rests almost all day, every day, relaxing and resting are much overdone. As Zak discovered, the need for movement that never gets satisfied will eventually feel like fatigue.

Moderate exercise will not wear you out, but sitting around too much will. And the cure for much of our fatigue may surprise you, as described in the next chapter.

51

What We Need Most for an Energy Boost

Quick quiz:

At what time of the day do you feel an energy lag and wish you had a quick boost?

- a. Early morning, upon rising?
- b. About noon?
- c. Mid-afternoon?
- d. Early evening, upon arriving home from work?
- e. After dinner, 7:00 to 8:00 pm?
- f. After a long commute by car or airplane?
- g. All of the above?

Based on the FDA's estimate that 80% of adults in the U.S. consume caffeine every day in search of a quick boost of energy,[63] many of you could have answered (g) All of the above.

The search for energy enhancement is universal. For the other 20% of the population, a common alternative to caffeine from coffee or soft drinks is a sugar rush from cookies, candy, or "energy bars" (which are really just higher priced candy bars). But a recent analysis of seventy research studies reached the conclusion that a much more

---

63. FDA (2007) "Caffeine and Your Body" *Understanding Over-the-Counter Medicines.* Available at http://www.fda.gov/downloads/Drugs/ResourcesForYou/Consumers/ BuyingUsingMedicineSafely/UnderstandingOver-the-CounterMedicines/UCM205286. pdf

effective energy boost is possible from a non-food source—physical exercise.[64]

A team at the University of Georgia exercise psychology laboratory found that 90% of the studies reviewed reached the same conclusion, that exercise increased energy and reduced fatigue. The physical exercise proved more effective than stimulants in drug form.

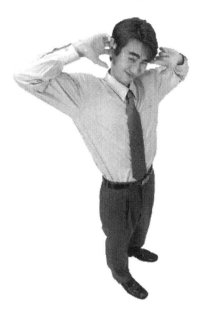

When interviewed, Dr. Patrick O'Connor admitted, "A lot of times when people are fatigued the last thing they want to do is exercise. But if you're physically inactive and fatigued, being just a bit more active will help."[65]

During any of the times listed in the Quick Quiz at the beginning of this chapter, physical exercise could provide the boost you are looking for to cure an energy lag.

A brisk walk in the morning can get you started even without a cup of coffee. During a long day at your desk, standing to stretch and walking to the water cooler can relieve the fatigue without a cola drink. After a long commute, or returning home after work, or just winding down after a long day, what your body is hungering for is movement, not more sitting.

64. Puetz, T., O'Connor, P., & Dishman, R., (2006) "Effects of Chronic Exercise on Feelings of Energy and Fatigue: A Quantitative Synthesis" *Psychological Bulletin,* 132(6) 866-876

65. Fahmy, S. (2007) "Regular Exercise Better Than Stimulants at Reducing Fatigue," *The University of Georgia Research Magazine,* Winter, 2007

52

Physical Activity is Part of Nutrition

IN 1992 THE USDA released its Food Guide Pyramid showing food groups in horizontal rows. The pyramid was updated in 2005 with many sleek changes, including vertical food group sections and most distinctively, a human figure walking up steps on the side.

In one discussion of why the changes were made, a person asked about the figure walking up the new pyramid and was told it represents the importance of exercise.

"Why was it not included in the original one? Was exercise not important then?"

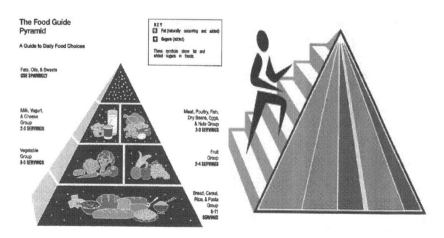

The answer: In 1992 the level of regular physical activity was significantly higher than in 2005. Before the earlier version, researchers assumed that exercise was a regular part of daily life so no visual reminder was needed. A great body of research completed after 1992 has uncovered the importance of exercise and the way sedentary lifestyles have been hurting our health.

Even in 2011 when the new pyramid was discontinued in favor of a new graphic, "Choose My Plate," the meal tracking worksheet with a suggested Daily Food Plan still shows Physical Activity in its own category, as if it were one of the food groups to be tracked.[66] The worksheet describes how much of each food group to eat and encourages adults to be active 150 minutes each week.

Contrary to food science studies of the past, physical activity has proven to be an essential aspect of human nutrition.

The importance of exercise to our nutritional state and health justifies its inclusion in this discussion of hungers, because so often the body's craving for movement is stifled with another snack or dessert. We continue to crave the novelty and recreation that exercise could be providing us.

The plethora of diet books and weight loss claims provides more evidence that the importance of exercise is being underestimated by the popular press. The next chapter addresses this obsession with weight loss and the scale, together with the absurd but popular notion that a person's weight is all-important.

---

66. http://www.choosemyplate.gov/food-groups/downloads/worksheets/ Worksheet_2000_18plusyr.pdf

53

Your Scale is Lying to You!

WHEN I WORKED in an Eating Disorders Unit many patients were obsessed with the scale. They came to the Unit for treatment because this preoccupation had reached a point of interfering with daily life and they were almost unable to function. Although these were extreme cases, I saw many attributes common to the thousands of "normal" men and women I have worked with before and since.

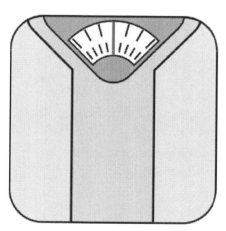

Many people are disturbed by the numbers on the scale. Like Diana, one of my Eating Disorders patients, they weigh themselves frequently and draw erroneous conclusions from what they see there.

At first, Diana noticed she was weighing herself daily. Eventually she began stepping on the scales several times a day. If I saw her in the morning and asked how she was, she would reply "I don't know how I am; I have not weighed myself yet." She gave the scale ultimate power over her mood and self-concept. If her weight had dipped slightly since yesterday, she was elated. If her weight had crept up, she was crushed, discouraged and depressed all day.

Diana's self-image depended on what the cruel scale told her.

When he was young, my brother-in-law came up with the idea that he wanted to cut his own hair. He hated barbers and didn't want to trouble his mother for haircutting money anyway. One day he got up early and found a pair of scissors. Too short to use the bathroom mirror, he found the toaster. He moved it close to the edge of the countertop and cut his hair by the reflection in the toaster.

Of course, the toaster was curved. What he saw was a funhouse mirror, not an accurate reflection. And his haircut?

It was so awful his mother took him to the barber on her way to work. It was an emergency!

While my father always said the difference between a good haircut and a bad one was three weeks, this doesn't apply when we're considering how our self-image is formed.

Like the curved mirror, the numbers on Diana's scale didn't convey an accurate image. The scale does not tell you what you think it is saying. All it can do is provide a single number that is affected by interactions of all the components of your body—how much water happens to be in your system, how much food has not been eliminated, how much muscle is burning glycogen for energy, how much fat is either being stored or being prepared for metabolism, and many other factors—but all those measures are combined in one overall number such that you have no idea what each of the components contributes. The conditions the scale is measuring can change from hour to hour.

Look at the description in the next chapter to see what is happening to two of those components that the scale is not revealing. I call them the Factory and the Warehouse.

54

Your Body's Factory and Warehouse

THE SCALE GIVES you only your weight. Another measure that researchers often use is BMI (Body Mass Index), but even that is an indicator of only height and weight and does not tell what is happening with fat stores and muscle mass within the body. Look at the following three graphics for a comparison of what happens in the body.

In the picture on the left, the shaded area represents Lean Body Mass (LBM or muscles and vital organs) and the white space represents fat storage. The center picture represents a body builder or someone with built-up muscles and very little fat storage. The picture on the right represents someone with minimal muscles but extra fat storage.

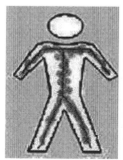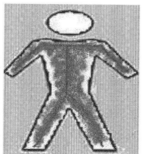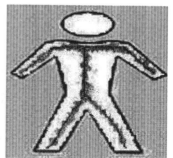

Note how the calorie requirements will be different for these three—the one in the center will need many more calories than the others to support all that muscle. And the one in the center will probably weigh more than the other two, even though the person is likely very healthy. The center one may even be thinner than the one on the right, while weighing more. Remember that what you weigh on the scale may be misleading about your health status.

The LBM is composed of the skeleton, vital organs, and muscle tissue. This is where energy is expended. Think of it as the *Factory* of the body where work gets done, where muscles constantly burn fuel for energy.

The greater your LBM, the more calories are required to keep it all going and your body functioning.

Your Body Fat is more like a *Warehouse*, where no work is being done and where no calories are being used. Its job is to store calories, not use them up, so it requires few if any calories to maintain.

The scale tells you nothing about what is going on in the Factory and Warehouse (LBM and Body Fat), but those are where the changes take place during the weight loss process. To understand these changes, note what happens to LBM and Body Fat when we track weight loss for a typical young woman.

This Case Study is a composite of dozens of women I have worked with. I will call her Cassie. She is an average female. At the start of the story she is 18 years old, 5'4" and weighs 120 lbs.

Total Weight	120 lbs.
Weight of LBM	90 lbs.
Weight of Body Fat	30 lbs.
Percent of LBM	75%
Percent of Body Fat	25%

Cassie is sports-minded and active all through high school. Her body fat is 25% which is a normal level for an adult female. Upon graduating, Cassie takes a desk job where she is *sedentary* and has no time for exercise. Sedentary means not physically active, the picture that comes to mind when you hear *couch potato*. Cassie is not being lazy; in fact, she is working hard at her desk, but she is sitting most of the day. Like most Americans, her life is characterized by sitting.

After a few years of her new sedentary life, Cassie finds she has gained twenty pounds. Starting with her original data, watch how it changes now. Instead of just looking at the weight she gained, notice what changed in her body as described on the chart.

Total Weight	120 lbs.	Gained 20 lbs.	140 lbs.
Weight of LBM	90 lbs.	LBM stayed the same	90 lbs.
Weight of Body Fat	30 lbs.	Gained 20 lbs. fat	50 lbs.
Percent of LBM	75%	LBM % went down	64%
Percent of Body Fat	25%	Fat % went up	36%

Since she has not been using her muscles actively, her LBM does not change. Her body fat is where the extra weight will be stored. Both fat pounds and fat percent have gone up.

The most typical reaction to this bad news from the scale is to try a crash diet. These are diets that promise fast weight loss—you can find them in nearly every woman's magazine on the newsstand. Despite the claims that you will lose amazing amounts without effort, there is no magic to these plans. After all, almost any extreme diet will cause weight loss by dramatically upsetting the body's equilibrium. Among the serious health problems they introduce is the imbalance of body fat these diets cause. Look how the chart of LBM changes with her new crash diet-induced weight loss.

Look closely at the numbers. Because the weight loss is so fast and extreme, the pounds come from her LBM, not from her fat stores. It is not biologically possible to burn the fat stores in a rapid crash diet.

As a typical busy woman, Cassie thinks she has no time to exercise but is in a hurry to get rid of the weight. Sadly, with no physical activity to burn any of the fat stores, even when she loses weight, the weight of her body fat stays the same. Her LBM percentage decreases and her body fat increases as a percent of the total.

Total Weight	120 lbs.	Lost 20 lbs. →	120 lbs.
Weight of LBM	90 lbs.	Lost LBM →	70 lbs.
Weight of Body Fat	30 lbs.	Fat stayed the same →	50 lbs.
Percent of LBM	75%	LBM % went down →	58%
Percent of Body Fat	25%	Fat % went up →	42%

This is the shocking result of the crash diet—even when she loses weight, she gains fat!

At this point the scale may show the same weight as she was originally (120), but the breakdown of LBM compared to fat has changed markedly, which will change many other things in her life. Most importantly, the LBM that used to burn more calories has shrunk so the Factory is smaller and has fewer calorie needs.

If Cassie is typical, at this point she will be thrilled with her weight loss, happy to be done with the crash diet, and eager to return to her former eating habits. Sadly, what used to be a normal calorie level for her original LBM is now too much for her smaller LBM. Eating what used to be normal is now too much and will quickly add more pounds to the Warehouse, her fat stores. This common rebound weight gain can be described with these additional changes on the chart.

Total Weight	120 lbs.	140 lbs.	120 lbs.	Gained 20 lbs. ⟶	140 lbs.
Weight of LBM	90 lbs.	90 lbs.	70 lbs.	LBM stayed same ⟶	70 lbs.
Weight of Body Fat	30 lbs.	50 lbs.	50 lbs.	Fat increased ⟶	70 lbs.
Percent of LBM	75%	64%	58%	LBM % went down ⟶	50%
Percent of Body Fat	25%	36%	42%	Fat % went up ⟶	50%

If she tries another extreme diet she will continue to gain fat even when she loses weight. Each time she goes through the cycle her calorie needs will decrease as the LBM proportion decreases.

This sad cycle of yo-yo dieting is very discouraging and worse each time—but it can be fixed!

To achieve a healthy weight loss, fat must be burned and LBM must be preserved or increased

All of these could help break the downward spiral:

- The most important ingredient in changing the cycle is physical activity. The CDC recommends 150 minutes per week of moderate exercise such as walking to maintain weight, or more to lose weight.[67]

---

67. http://www.cdc.gov/physicalactivity/everyone/health/#ControlWeight

- The process must be gradual in order to successfully burn fat.

- She needs to eat sufficient calories so the body does not feel deprived and compelled to conserve by storing more fat.

- She needs balanced nutrition so the LBM can be built up with the necessary vitamins, minerals, and proteins.

- She needs sufficient carbohydrates to support the energy-burning cycle, including complex carbs (fiber) for satiety.

- She should be careful not to skip meals to avoid deprivation feelings.

More Bad News about Crash Diets

Before following any new eating plan, especially one promoted with expensive treatments, drinks, equipment, and/or supplements, you need to think seriously about the possible long-term consequences. High protein diets put extra strain on the kidneys, and very low calorie diets can cause serious nutrient deficiencies. To show a temporary weight loss, stresses are placed on many organ systems that are all affected by a major nutritional shift.

I have researched hundreds of different diets, some with intriguing and tantalizing names: the Ice Cream Diet, the Cookie Diet, the Three Hour Diet, the Milkshake Diet—what won't they think of next?

People frequently ask me, "Does this diet *work*?" I can answer truthfully—yes and no.

Yes. Just about anything out there could work in the sense that your nutritional balance will be so disturbed that you will probably lose weight initially. Your LBM will probably suffer as in Cassie's example above, but *yes*, you could actually lose weight on even the craziest eating plan.

But, no. It will not work in the sense of being healthy for your body, making you feel strong and energetic, or maintaining the weight loss. The best way to test the effectiveness of any eating plan is to ask yourself:

- How do you feel while you are following the diet?

- Do you have energy for normal daily activities and fun physical recreation?

- Do you sleep well?

- Does the plan allow a good balance of protein, carbs, and healthy fats?

- Is it a plan you can comfortably follow for years at a time?

~ 55 ~

The Alternative to Diets

MOST AMERICANS DO *not* need a diet to follow. Instead they need to eat a healthy variety of foods they enjoy, and they need to feed all their hungers in ways that preserve health and leave them feeling satisfied.

If you want to look for people with an extensive body of real-world evidence about what works to lose weight *and keep it off permanently,* then you will be interested in the National Weight Control Registry (NWCR). Initiated by Rena Wing and James Hill, both renowned obesity researchers, NWCR is a collection of real personal experiences from adults with long-term weight loss experience.

The minimum for eligibility to join is at least thirty pounds lost with the loss maintained for more than a year. And this is not just a handful of participants in a small study—the registry numbers over 5,000 members who, on average, have lost 66 pounds and kept it off for over five years. They share stories, not hyped up marketing messages, but stories from regular people who are weight loss experts because they have experienced the remarkable changes personally.

Of the Registry participants, 94% reported that their success was partly due to increasing their physical activity.[68] They did not all report expensive gym memberships or complicated workout routines, in fact, the activity that worked for most was walking, and 90% reported they exercise about an hour each day.

---

68. http://www.nwcr.ws/Research/default.htm

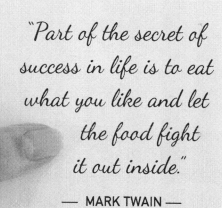

"Part of the secret of
success in life is to eat
what you like and let
the food fight
it out inside."

— MARK TWAIN —

56

Time for Your Activity Recess!

IN ONE OF MY nutrition classes, as students learned about the negative health effects of the couch potato and snacking lifestyle, one man grew concerned about his younger brother. He posed a question to the class: "How can I motivate my brother who is very overweight?"

Students responded with wonderfully creative suggestions along the general theme of these ideas:

- Start small and be involved personally.

- Invite him to go on a hike with you.

- Connect to another hobby or interest he has.

- Try Geo-Caching! It is a game with a GPS that makes you hike around to find landmarks.[69]

- If he is into video games, try the Wii Sports Resort.

- Xbox Kinect games can get your heart pumping.

- Shoot some hoops together.

- Get him a dog to take for runs or walks.

---

69. See www.geocaching.com

- Don't let on that it is "exercise," but let him think it is something just for fun!

As these students had discovered, people react differently if exercise is another burdensome duty to squeeze into an already burdened life. But we are all more likely to jump at the chance of taking a fun break if it is for recreation. The trick is to think of *active* recreation pursuits.

As we did when we were in grade school, take a break from your desk job or your studies and call it your *recess!* Keep in mind the mental picture of kids shouting for joy as they burst out on to the playground and leave your desk for an Activity Recess.

Your own Activity Recess will be most fun if you tailor it closely to your own personality and favorites. I may not want to shoot some hoops but my husband can't resist that. My 90-year-old mother may not want a killer-robot Xbox game, but she loves Wii tennis and bowling.

What is your favorite?

Remember when you feel like eating that you may be hungry for something other than that snack or extra dessert. Maybe your body is telling you it craves the novelty of movement, recreation, and physical activity.

57

FingerTIPS about the Hunger for Novelty

- Many people eat out of boredom or when they crave novelty, but the food fix is temporary and not what the body really needs.

- Our modern sedentary lifestyles have led to deficiencies in physical activity that harm our health and for which we need to find creative solutions.

- Our bones, joints, and circulatory systems crave movement, especially given the sedentary lifestyles our modern conveniences provide.

- Moderate physical exercise can provide an energy boost and relieve fatigue.

- Any discussion of nutrition must include physical activity as a critical part of a person's nutritional status.

- Obsessions with weight loss instead of health lead to preoccupation with numbers on the scale. Our weight is a poor indicator of body composition.

- Healthy weight loss is slow and gradual, and it preserves lean body mass.

- One way to find the novelty your body hungers for is by taking an Activity Recess, where you choose a physical activity that is fun and meets your own unique definition of recreation.

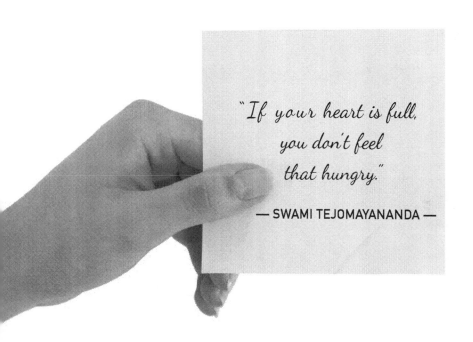

"*If your heart is full,
you don't feel
that hungry.*"

— SWAMI TEJOMAYANANDA —

58

Resources about Fitness and Exercise

A PANEL OF EXPERTS discussing fitness was once asked, "Which is the *best* exercise?" A lively discussion followed with some arguing for swimming (exercises all muscles in the body), walking (easiest to do, needs no special equipment), and many others. Finally the moderator interrupted with, "There's one clear winner for the *very best* exercise. That is . . . whatever exercise you will actually *do!*"

I agree that moving your body in any way that you will enjoy enough to keep it up regularly will be the best exercise program for you. If you want fitness guides to give ideas and specific exercise guidance, look for books recommended by healthcare professionals you trust.

Following are just the tip of the iceberg of some I have used, which you may explore for more information as you become more aware of the fifth hunger for novelty and movement.

Hutchinson, Alex, (2011), *Which Comes First, Cardio or Weights? Fitness Myths, Training Truths, and Other Surprising Discoveries from the Science of Exercise*, Harper Collins, New York

> This book covers the full spectrum of exercise science with helpful diagrams and practical tips on using proven science to improve fitness and reach weight loss goals.

Nelson, Miriam, (1998), *Strong Women Stay Slim* Bantam

Dr. Nelson's original book, *Strong Women Stay Young,* explained why strength training helps beat the aging process. This guide follows in that tradition, with reliable information about the exercise needed for most effective weight loss.

Dahm, Diane & Smith, Jay, (2005), *Mayo Clinic Fitness for Everybody,* Mayo Clinic, Minnesota

A detailed guide to getting and staying fit for all ages and conditions. Illustrations and guides make it practical and easy-to-follow without expensive equipment.

Bailey, Covert, (2000), *The Ultimate Fit or Fat: An all-new program to get you in shape and keep you in shape*

One of the great classics in exercise books, *Fit or Fat* from the 1970s was updated in 2000 and is still reliable and motivating.

Christensen, Alice, (2002), *The American Yoga Association's Beginner's Manual: The Definitive Guide from the Nation's Preeminent Yoga Center,* Fireside, New York

Includes three 10-week programs of exercise with clear instructions and photos. Invites you to use yoga techniques to improve health and become happier with yourself and with the challenges of daily life.

✢ 59 ✢

FingerFOODS
Recipe for the Fifth Hunger

WHEN YOU ARE hungering for novelty, don't fall for the media pressure to open a boring bag of chips or crackers. This colorful salsa is ultra-low-fat and packed with healthy fiber, protein, and phytochemicals. Eat it with cucumber slices.

The bright colors and novel flavor combinations will energize you for a brisk walk with a friend.

Fiesta Black Bean Salsa

2 cups cooked black beans
   (1 16-oz can or cook from dry beans)
2 cups sweet corn, canned, frozen, or fresh
1 cup chopped green bell pepper
1 cup chopped red bell pepper
1 cup chopped yellow bell pepper
1 cup grated carrots
½ cup chopped cilantro (optional)
2 cups of your favorite salsa, bottled or made fresh

Drain and rinse beans and corn. Combine with chopped and grated vegetables. Add cilantro if desired. Will keep longer in refrigerator without added salsa, which can be added right before serving. Can be used as a salad, dip, or side dish.

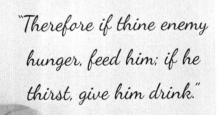

"Therefore if thine enemy hunger, feed him; if he thirst, give him drink."

— ROMANS 12:20 —

‑ PART VI ‑

The Whole Hand

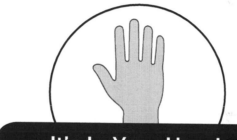

It's In Your Hands

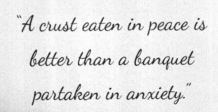

"A crust eaten in peace is
better than a banquet
partaken in anxiety."

— AESOP —

60

The Whole Hand

Now that you have seen all the fingers and the hungers they represent, they can form your portable nutrition calculator as described in Chapter 5. Here is a sample of how it can work.

Tim is trying to eat healthier. One afternoon he finds himself thinking about getting a burger and fries because it is a habit he has followed for years without thinking. He stops to do the *Five Hunger Check*.

He starts with his thumb (see Part 1), and decides whether his blood sugar has been well-controlled with evenly spaced meals today (see Chapters 8 and 11).

If he realizes he has not been eating at moderate intervals, he has a sensible snack to even out his blood sugar level (see Chapter 14). If he decides meals have been well moderated, he goes on to his index finger.

For the second hunger (see Part 2), Tim uses his index finger to remember how to measure his satiety index (see Chapter 20). If the number is 2.5 or less, he recognizes it is time to eat and looks for food with low energy density (see Chapter 21) and high nutrient density (see Chapter 22). Or if his satiety measures 3 or more, he realizes this hunger is already satisfied and goes on to the next finger.

For the third hunger (see Part 3), Tim thinks about his middle finger and checks his emotional state (see Chapter 32). If there are emotional cues he recognizes, then he plans some healthy comfort foods (see Chapter 37) or meets his emotional needs in alternate ways (see Chapter 33). If after the Emotional Hunger Checklist he concludes it is not an emotional need, he proceeds to the next finger.

The ring finger helps Tim think about his fourth hunger, concerning stability and habits (see Part 4). He reviews why he is craving a burger and fries (see Chapter 41), the habits he has grown accustomed to and his food environment (see Chapter 46). If he realizes he has developed habits that are leading him in unhealthy directions, he considers what it will take to make a change (see Chapter 45). If he decides his hunger is not related to habits, he moves on to the next finger.

For the fifth hunger (see Part 5), Tim uses his pinky to consider his need for novelty. He thinks about his daily routine and realizes he has been sitting all day and would really welcome a chance to stretch and get fresh air. Instead of his original plan to stop for fast food, he decides to go for a bike ride along the new parkway near his home. When he is done he feels refreshed and energized and realizes he does not want the burger and fries after all.

Later that afternoon, Tim remembers his index finger again and checks his satiety one more time. Now he is feeling a little empty, about a 2 (see Chapter 20), so he is ready for a healthy dinner that he enjoys heartily.

It's in our hands.

"There are people in
the world so hungry, that
God cannot appear to them
except in the form
of bread."

— MAHATMA GANDHI —

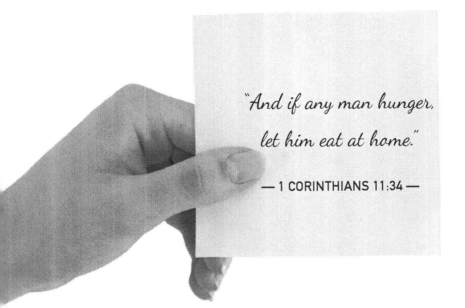

"And if any man hunger,

let him eat at home."

— 1 CORINTHIANS 11:34 —

✢ PART VII ✢

Appendix

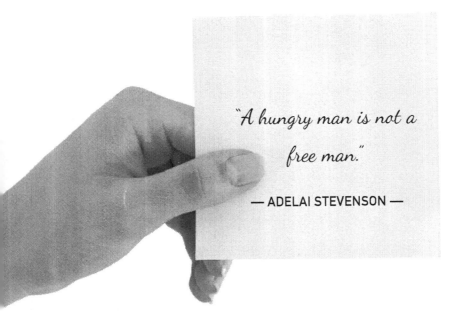

"A hungry man is not a free man."

— ADELAI STEVENSON —

61

WORLD HUNGER:
Why are people still hungry?

FOR TOO MANY people in the world, the Five Hungers system might seem an absurd luxury because they face bone-deep true hunger every day of their lives. In 2010, the United Nations announced there were almost one billion hungry people in the world, which is about one in every seven people. In this context, "hunger" means protein-energy malnutrition, or the lack of both protein for growth and enough calories to sustain life.[70]

Children's hunger is most serious, as it makes every childhood disease worse and leads to five million deaths per year. Another child dies of hunger every six seconds, which is how long it took you to read this sentence.[71]

The world produces enough food that we need not have any hungry people at all. We produce enough food for each person in the world to have over 2700 calories per day.[72] We just can't match the supply with the demand.

Why are so many people still hungry? The primary reason is

---

70. 2012 *World Hunger and Poverty Facts and Statistics from World Hunger Education Service,* available at http://www.worldhunger.org/articles/Learn/world%20hunger%20facts%20 2002.htm#Footnotes
71. Bryce, J., Boschi-Pinto, C., Shibuya, K., Black, R. and the WHO Child Health Epidemiology Reference Group (2005), "WHO estimates of the causes of death in children." *Lancet* ; 365: 1147–52

poverty. In many areas, people are poor because they can't grow food due to lack of water, land, or stability. People who subsist on less than $2 a day simply can't afford to buy food. Even if they could, in many developing countries the infrastructure is inadequate to get food where it is needed.

A second cause is armed conflict. War keeps people hungry and in poverty and was the cause of 36 million people displaced as refugees either internally or exiled at the end of 2008.[73] Many other causes including climate change may be contributing to the overall picture of poverty and, in turn, hunger.[74]

---

72. Food and Agriculture Organization, International Fund for Agricultural Development, World Food Program, (2002) "Reducing Poverty and Hunger, the Critical Role of Financing for Food, Agriculture, and Rural Development"

73. UNHCR 2008 Global Report (2008) "The Year in Review" *United Nations High Commissioner for Refugees,* available at http://www.unhcr.org/4a2d0b1d2.pdf

74. See *Climate change, global warming and the effect on poor people,* available at http://www. worldhunger.org/env_hunger.htm#global warming

62

What Can Be Done about World Hunger?

IT IS IMPORTANT that we not forget the truly hungry in our privileged and sometimes oblivious lives. Even in the U.S. about 16 million people (one in every 19) experience "very low food security."[75]

World hunger is not inevitable; it can be alleviated. Hundreds of organizations are actively working to do just that. Some successes have already been won; in fact progress has been made in Asia, Latin America, and the Caribbean. But elsewhere in the world hunger has grown worse in recent years. More can be done, and individuals can help.

The United Nations' World Food Programme (WFP) calls hunger *the world's No. 1 health risk and the world's greatest solvable problem.*[76] The two most important ways that the World Hunger Education Service (WHES) believes individuals can make a difference in world hunger are to understand the scope and nature of the problem, and to take action.

If you are involved in education, you are invited to include topics on world hunger when you teach. Classroom activities and extensive curricula are provided on the WFP Web site.[77] They even sponsor an online game called *Free Rice* where participants learn about hunger

---

75. http://feedingamerica.org/hunger-in-america/hunger-facts/hunger-and-poverty-statis-tics.aspx
76. http://www.wfp.org/hunger/greatest-solvable-problem
77. http://www.wfp.org/students-and-teachers/teachers

(and other general education topics) and simply by playing, enable donations of rice by the Web site sponsors to be used by WFP.[78] What could be more rewarding than feeding people by playing a game?

Action can take the form of donating to relief organizations, lobbying for policy changes, and working directly with hungry people. Excellent resources and links to find an activity that fits for you can be found on the WHES Web site.[79]

People can find great satisfaction in sharing their abundance with the less fortunate, and there are unlimited ways to do it. One example is the Church of Jesus Christ of Latter-day Saints (the "Mormons") who promote a day of fasting every month, after which members are encouraged to donate the value of food not eaten to relieve needs in their communities and elsewhere in the world.[80]

Almost 800,000 people work on alleviating poverty by participating in micro-loan programs such as Kiva.[81]

The WFP also invites people to join their online community to fight hunger. Estimating that two billion people use the internet and one billion are hungry, their *Billion for a Billion* program seeks to harness online time and resources from the haves to help the have-nots. You can see their programs, many choices of how you can help and more information about world hunger on their *Fighting Hunger Worldwide* site.[82]

As you consider your own hunger, pause to also think of your starving brothers and sisters around the world. Spending time learning about world hunger and getting involved with efforts to help are two great ways to feed your own emotional hunger (see Part 3) and feel good about yourself.

---

78. http://freerice.com/about/faq
79. http://www.worldhunger.org/reduce.htm
80. See http://www.lds.org/study/topics/fasting-and-fast-offerings?lang=eng
81. http://www.kiva.org/
82. http://www.wfp.org/get-involved/ways-to-help

63

My Favorite Books

I'VE BEEN WORKING in nutrition and health for four decades and during that time I've read thousands of pages (paper and electronic) on the topic. The overwhelming amount of information available prompted me to find a way to make sense of it all and then to formulate an easy-to-remember system to help people (myself included!) remember why I'm really eating.

Hence, the 5 Hungers and the Five Fingers system.

However, many people ask me what I think of this or that book, diet, website, etc., so I'm going to give you a selection if you want to study these topics in more detail.

Resources about Blood Sugar

American Diabetes Association, *MyFoodAdvisor: Recipes for Healthy Living,* available at http://bit.ly/myfoodadvisor

A free online resource with recipes, cooking tips and a meal plan to follow; appropriate for those managing diabetes and anyone interested in controlling blood sugar. Registering online (free) gives access to daily meal plans, recipes and other tools.

Fries, Wendy C., (2011), "13 Ways to Fight Sugar Cravings," *WebMD Feature,* available at http://bit.ly/fightcravings

Ideas and tips for sensible and healthy ways to deal with cravings.

Fittante, Ann, (2006), *The Sugar Solution: Your Symptoms are Real and Your Solution is Here,* Prevention Magazine

Tools to identify and correct high blood sugar and drop excess pounds, replenish energy stores, and reduce disease risk.

Kessler, David A., (2009), T*he End of Overeating: Taking Control of the Insatiable American Appetite,* Rodale, New York

Describes the way the food industry designs, manufactures, advertises and distributes foods that stimulate our appetites to the point we lose control over our eating habits.

Pollan, Michael, (2006), *The Omnivore's Dilemma: A Natural History of Four Meals,* Penguin Press, New York

Provides answers to the question "What should we have for dinner?" by examining in detail where our food comes from, comparing natural to processed foods.

Resources about Physical Emptiness

Rolls, Barbara, (2012), *The Ultimate Volumetrics Diet: Smart, Simple, Science-Based Strategies for Losing Weight and Keeping It Off,* Harper Collins, New York

Suggests eating plans based on low energy density, so you can fill up on more foods.

Ornish, Dean, (2000), *Eat More, Weigh Less: Dr. Dean Ornish's Life Choice Program for Losing Weight Safely While Eating Abundantly,* Harper Collins, New York

> Takes the approach of abundance rather than deprivation to lose weight and reduce risk for cancer and other chronic diseases.

Nutritiondata.com, *The Fullness Factor*, available at http://nutritiondata.self.com/topics/fullness-factor

> Gives a predicted level of satiety to common foods based on a mathematical formula and the ingredient content.

Zinczenko, David and Goulding, Matt, (2011), *Eat This, Not That! The No-Diet Weight Loss Solution*, Rodale, New York

> Editors of *Men's Health* magazine distill diet decisions down to simple comparisons between foods with high energy density compared to better choices, with colorful photos of common fast food meals and favorite foods.

Groger, M. & Lebherz, T., (1985), *Eating Awareness Training: The Natural Way to Permanent Weight Loss,* Simon & Schuster, New York

> This book presents a six-week program to teach awareness of when your body has enough, protect yourself from an unhealthy urge to eat, and be free from diets and calorie counting.

Resources about Emotional Eating

Mayo Clinic, (2009), *Weight Loss Help: Gain Control of Emotional Eating,* available at http://www.mayoclinic.com/health/weight-loss/MH00025

Describes how emotional eating can sabotage your weight-loss efforts and provides tips to regain control of your eating habits.

Van Hart, Zach, *Get a Handle on Emotional Eating: The Secret Sabotage of Your Program,* by SparkPeople®, available at http://www.sparkpeople.com

Harding, Ann, (2011) "Study Offers Clues to Emotional Eating," CNN Health, available at http://www.cnn.com/2011/HEALTH/07/25/study.clues.emotional.eating/index.html

Psychology Today, "*Emotional Eating Test*"

Interactive test with 149 questions, partial results free, full results with personalized interpretation available for purchase at http://psychologytoday.tests.psychtests.com

Hatfield, Heather, (2003), "Emotional Eating: Feeding Your Feelings," Eating to feed a feeling, and not a growling stomach, is emotional eating, WebMD Feature, available at http://www.webmd.com/diet/features/emotional-eating-feeding-your-feelings

Tribole, Evelyn & Resch Elyse, (2003), *Intuitive Eating: A Revolutionary Program That Works,* St Martin's Press

Intuitive Eating focuses on nurturing your body rather than starving it, encourages natural weight loss, and helps you find the weight you were meant to be.

Resources about Habit Change

Aldana, Steven, (2005), *The Culprit and the Cure: Why Lifestyle Is the Culprit Behind America's Poor Health,* Maple Mountain Press

> Explains in a light-hearted but scientifically supported way how the average person can make effective lifestyle changes in diet and exercise.

Claiborn, James & Pedrick, Cherry, (2001), *The Habit Change Workbook: How to Break Bad Habits and Form Good Ones,* New Harbinger Publications, Oakland, CA

> This step-by-step, cognitive-behavioral program helps you break unwanted habits and replace them with healthy new ones. This book has been awarded The Association for Behavioral and Cognitive Therapies Self-Help Seal of Merit.

Duhigg, Charles, (2012), *The Power of Habit: Why We Do What We Do in Life and Business,* Random House, New York

> Combines research and stories about how habits shape our lives and how we can shape our habits.

Heath, Chip & Heath, Dan, (2010), *Switch: How to Change Things When Change Is Hard,* Broadway Books, New York

> The Heaths bring together research in psychology, sociology, and other fields about how we can effect transformative change. Switch shows that successful changes follow a pattern you can use in changing the world or changing your waistline.

Ryan, M.J., (2006), *This Year I Will . . . . How to Finally Change a Habit, Keep a Resolution, or Make a Dream Come True,* Broadway Books, New York

Describes the secret to making changes that stick. Breakthrough wisdom and coaching to help readers make this time the time that change becomes permanent.

Selig, Meg, (2009), *Changepower!: 37 Secrets to Habit Change Success,* Taylor & Francis, New York

A step-by-step process to achieve any habit change goal. First-person stories, pithy quotes, and how-to exercises provide inspiration, humor, and encouragement as readers embark on their habit change journeys.

Resources about Fitness and Exercise

Hutchinson, Alex, (2011), *Which Comes First, Cardio or Weights? Fitness Myths, Training Truths, and Other Surprising Discoveries from the Science of Exercise,* Harper Collins, New York

Covers the full spectrum of exercise science with helpful diagrams and practical tips on using proven science to improve fitness and reach weight loss goals.

Nelson, Miriam, (1998), *Strong Women Stay Slim,* Bantam

Dr. Nelson's original book, *Strong Women Stay Young,* explained why strength training helps beat the aging process. This guide follows in that tradition with reliable information about the exercise needed for most effective weight loss.

Dahm, Diane & Smith, Jay, (2005), *Mayo Clinic Fitness for Everybody,* Mayo Clinic, Minnesota

A detailed guide to getting and staying fit for all ages and conditions. Illustrations and guides make is practical and easy-to-follow without expensive equipment.

Bailey, Covert, (2000), *The Ultimate Fit or Fat: An all-new program to get you in shape and keep you in shape*

> One of the great classics in exercise books, *Fit or Fat,* from the 1970s was updated in 2000 and is still reliable and motivating.

Christensen, Alice, (2002), *The American Yoga Association's Beginner's Manual: The Definitive Guide from the Nation's Preeminent Yoga Center,* Fireside, New York

> Includes three 10-week programs of exercise with clear instructions and photos. Invites you to use yoga techniques to improve health and become happier with yourself and with the challenges of daily life.

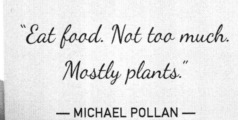

"Eat food. Not too much.
Mostly plants."

— MICHAEL POLLAN —

References

1. Twain, M. (1880) *A Tramp Abroad*, available at Project Gutenberg

2. Twain, M., (1897) *Following the Equator: A Journey around the World*, Chapter 43, American Publishing Co., Hartford, CT

3. http://www.huffingtonpost.com/dr-dean-ornish/globalization-of-illnessg_b_558.html

4. Janssen, I., (2007) "Morbidity and mortality risk associated with an overweight BMI in older men and women." *Obesity* (Silver Spring). 2007 Jul;15(7):1827-40.

    Zajacova, J. & Burgard, S. (2011) "Overweight Adults May Have the Lowest Mortality—Do They Have the Best Health?" *American Journal of Epidemiology.* 173(4) 430-437.

5. http://www.ers.usda.gov/publications/aer833/aer833.pdf

6. http://www.ncbi.nlm.nih.gov/books/NBK22436/

7. Bauer, H. & Matthews, K. (2012) *Bread Is the Devil: Win the weight loss battle by taking control of your diet demons.* St. Martin's Press. New York.

8. http://www.fruitsandveggiesmatter.gov/index.html

9. Brownell, K., Popkin, B., et al (2009) "The Public Health and Economic Benefits of Taxing Sugar-Sweetened Beverages," *New England Journal of Medicine* 361(16):1599-1605.

10. http://www.yaleruddcenter.org/what_we_do.aspx?id=98

11. Tucker, K et al, (2006) "Colas, but not other carbonated beverages, are associated with low bone mineral density in older women: The Framingham Osteoporosis Study," *American Journal of Clinical Nutrition* 84(4) 936-942.

12. http://www.sugarstacks.com/

13. Higgins, J., Tuttle, T., Higgins, C., (2010) "Energy Beverages: Content and Safety" *Mayo Clinic Proceedings.* 85(11): 1033-41.

14. Brody, J. (2011) "Scientists See Dangers in Energy Drinks" *The New York Times*, 31 January 2011.

15. Taylor, R. (2008) "Red Bull drink lifts stroke risk: Australian Study" *Reuters* 14 August 2008

16. Winston, P. et al (2005) "Neuropsychiatric effects of caffeine." *Advances in Psychiatric Treatment* 11:432-439.

17. Kovacs, B. "What are the sources of caffeine," *Caffeine. MedicineNet.com* Available at http://www.medicinenet.com/caffeine/article.htm

18. Ibid.

19. Juliano, L.M., and R.R. Griffiths. "A Critical Review of Caffeine Withdrawal: Empirical Validation of Symptoms and Signs, Incidence, Severity, and Associated Features." *Psychopharmacology* (Berl). Sept, 21, 2004.

20. Varies with bottling location, sometimes does not contain caffeine; check label.

21. See http://www.drmcdougall.com

22. http://courses.cornell.edu/content.php?catoid=12&navoid=2188

23. http://www.nabiscoworld.com/oreo/

24. Pollan, M., (2006) *The Omnivore's Dilemma: A Natural History of Four Meals,* The Penguin Press, New York, page 3.

25. Euromonitor International, cited in http://www.nationmaster.com/graph/foo_sof_dri_con-food-soft-drink-consumption#source

26. See http://www.sleepfoundation.org/

27. Thorpy, M. (2003) "Sleep Hygiene" Ask the Expert, National Sleep Foundation. Available at http://www.sleepfoundation.org/article/ask-the-expert/sleep-hygiene.

28. American Academy of Pediatrics. Policy Statement. "The Use and Misuse of Fruit Juice in Pediatrics" *Pediatrics* 107 (5) May 2001, 1210-1213.

29. Thorpy, M. (2003) "Sleep Hygiene" Ask the Expert, National Sleep Foundation. Available at http://www.sleepfoundation.org/article/ask-the-expert/sleep-hygiene.

30. Wu, H.W. & Sturm, R. "What's on the menu? A review of the energy and nutritional content of U.S. chain restaurant menus" *Public Health Nutrition,* 2012, May 11:1-10.

31. Benoit, S.C. et al. (2009) "Palmitic acid mediates hypothalamic insulin resistance" *The Journal of Clinical Investigation,* 119:9

32. Groger, M. & Lebherz, T. (1985) *Eating Awareness Training: The Natural Way to Permanent Weight Loss* Simon & Schuster: New York.

33. Nutritional data and wheat label image courtesy of www.NutritionData.com .

34. Bread label and bread label image courtesy of www.wonderbread.com .

35. Fuhrman, J. "Nutrient Density," Available at http://www.drfuhrman.com/library/article17.aspx

36. http://www.eatrightamerica.com/erni-superfoods

37. Holt, S.H.A., et al (1995) "A satiety index of common foods" *European Journal of Clinical Nutrition,* 49: 675-690.

38. McCall Smith, A. (2009) *The Miracle at Speedy Motors, A No. 1 Ladies' Detective Agency* Novel, Random House.

39. For a start, see http://www.fruitcarving.com/ and http://www.foodgarnishing.com/id27.html

40. Davis, C., Strachan, S., Berkson, M. (2004) "Sensitivity to reward: implications for overeating and overweight" *Appetite,* 42 (2) 131-138.

41. Ibid.

42. Van Oudenhove, L. et al, (2011) "Fatty acid–induced gut-brain signaling attenuates neural and behavioral effects of sad emotion in humans." *Journal of Clinical Investigation.* 121(8):3094–3099.

43. Patel, K.A., & Schlundt, D.G. (2001) "Impact of Moods and Social Context on Eating Behavior, Appetite. 36(2) p 111-118.

44. Harvard Mental Health Letter, "Why stress causes people to overeat" February 2012. Available at http://www.health.harvard.edu/newsletters/Harvard_Mental_Health_Letter/2012/February/why-stress-causes-people-to-overeat

45. Available at http://www.heart.org/HEARTORG/GettingHealthy/StressManagement/FightStressWithHealthyHabits/Fight-Stress-with-Healthy-Habits_UCM_307992_Article.jsp

46. Available at office.microsoft.com/en-us/templates/food-diary-TC006089420.aspx

47. Ratey, J. (2008) *Spark: The Revolutionary New Science of Exercise and the Brain.* Little, Brown and Company, New York.

48. Raglin, J.S (1990) "Exercise and mental health. Beneficial and detrimental effects" Sports Medicine 9(6): 323-9.

49. Moll, J. (2006) "Human fronto–mesolimbic networks guide decisions about charitable donation" *Proceedings of the National Academy of Sciences.* 103 (42) 15623-8.

50. Farino, L. "Do Good, Feel Good: New research shows that helping others may be the key to happiness" *MSN Health.* Available at http://health.msn.com/health-topics/depression/do-good-feel-good

51. http://www.helpothers.org

52. http://www.kiva.org/lend

53. http://www.randomactsofkindness.org/

54. http://www.helpothers.org/story.php?sid=31133

55. USDA Available at http://ndb.nal.usda.gov/ndb/foods/show/7534

56. Miller, J. (2008) "Frybead: This seemingly simple food is a complicated symbol in Navajo culture" *Smithsonian Magazine* July, 2008. Available at http://www.smithsonianmag.com/people-places/frybread.html#ixzz1vTPPViTM

57. CDC (2003) *MMWR Weekly* August 1, 2003 / 52(30);702-704. Available at http://www.cdc.gov/mmwr/preview/mmwrhtml/mm5230a3.htm

58. Spurlock, M. (2004) *Super Size Me.* Morgan Spurlock Projects. Available at http://morganspurlock.com/super-size-me/

59. New York City Department of Health and Mental Hygiene, "Cutting Salt, Improving Health." Available at http://www.nyc.gov/html/doh/html/cardio/cardio-salt-initiative.shtml

60. Grunburg, M., (2010) *The Habit Factor®: An Innovative Method to Align Habits with Goals to Achieve Success,* Equilibrium Enterprises, La Jolla, CA.

61. Heath, C. and Heath D., (2010) *Switch: How to Change Things When Change Is Hard.* Broadway Books, New York.

62. Grontved, A. & Hu, F. "Television Viewing and Risk of Type 2 Diabetes, Cardiovascular Disease, and All-Cause Mortality: A Meta-analysis" *Journal of the American Medical Association* 305(23):2448-2455.

63. FDA (2007) "Caffeine and Your Body" *Understanding Over-the-Counter Medicines.* Available at http://www.fda.gov/downloads/Drugs/ResourcesForYou/Consumers/BuyingUsingMedicineSafely/UnderstandingOver-the-CounterMedicines/UCM205286.pdf

64. Puetz, T., O'Connor, P., & Dishman, R., (2006) "Effects of Chronic Exercise on Feelings of Energy and Fatigue: A Quantitative Synthesis" *Psychological Bulletin.* 132(6) 866-876.

65. Fahmy, S. (2007) "Regular Exercise Better Than Stimulants at Reducing Fatigue," *The University of Georgia Research Magazine,* Winter, 2007.

66. http://www.choosemyplate.gov/food-groups/downloads/worksheets/Worksheet_2000_18plusyr.pdf

67. http://www.cdc.gov/physicalactivity/everyone/health/#ControlWeight

68. http://www.nwcr.ws/Research/default.htm

69. See www.geocaching.com

70. 2012 World Hunger and Poverty Facts and Statistics from World Hunger Education Service, Available at http://www.worldhunger.org/articles/Learn/world%20hunger%20facts%202002.htm#Footnotes

71. Bryce, J., Boschi-Pinto, C., Shibuya, K., Black, R. and the WHO Child Health

Epidemiology Reference Group (2005). "WHO estimates of the causes of death in children." Lancet ; 365: 1147–52.

72. Food and Agriculture Organization, International Fund for Agricultural Development, World Food Program. (2002) "Reducing Poverty and Hunger, the Critical Role of Financing for Food, Agriculture, and Rural Development."

73. UNHCR 2008 Global Report (2008) "The Year in Review" United Nations High Commissioner for Refugees. Available at http://www.unhcr.org/4a2d0b1d2.pdf

74. See Climate change, global warming and the effect on poor people Available at http://www.worldhunger.org/env_hunger.htm#global warming

75. http://feedingamerica.org/hunger-in-america/hunger-facts/hunger-and-poverty-statistics.aspx

76. http://www.wfp.org/hunger/greatest-solvable-problem

77. http://www.wfp.org/students-and-teachers/teachers

78. http://freerice.com/about/faq

79. http://www.worldhunger.org/reduce.htm

80. See http://www.lds.org/study/topics/fasting-and-fast-offerings?lang=eng

81. http://www.kiva.org/

82. http://www.wfp.org/get-involved/ways-to-help

⊰ 65 ⊱

FingerTIPS

Summaries of the most important take-home messages for each of the five hungers are provided on the following pages so you can tear them out and keep them handy.

THE FIRST HUNGER

"Thumbnail" Sketch of Managing Blood Sugar

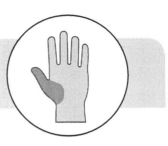

- A hectic lifestyle may be keeping you from healthy blood sugar levels if you skip breakfast, go for long periods without eating, then eat high-sugar and high-fat meals.

- Low blood sugar often causes fatigue and carbohydrate cravings.

- Carbohydrates are not the enemy and are an important part of a healthy diet.

- The simplest carbs are sugars that digest quickly

- Starch is made of many simple sugars connected in the same molecule.

- Fiber is the most complex carb, made of thousands of simple sugars. It lasts longer in the digestive tract so your blood sugar does not dip as fast.

- Soft drinks are a common way of taking in too many sugars quickly without getting filled up. Fruit juices are better but still should be limited since they are also high in sugar. Even better is a whole piece of fruit.

- Caffeine is a stimulant that can give the feeling of energy, but tolerance and adaptation develop quickly. It is easy to overuse caffeine.

- White flour is a refined carb that digests quickly and does not keep blood sugar as level as whole grains and other foods high in complex carbs (fiber).

- Evenly-spaced meals will help control blood sugar. Try to go no longer than five hours between meals or schedule a small snack if the interval will be longer than five hours.

- Foods that will help control blood sugar include more complex carbs and fewer sugars, eaten together with proteins and healthy fats.

- Take the Diabetes Risk Test to see if you need to consult your healthcare provider about your blood sugar control.

THE SECOND HUNGER

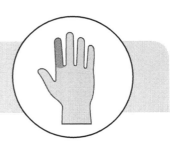

Index Finger:
Hunger of Physical Emptiness

- Rate your physical hunger by concentrating on a point in the center of your abdomen and assign a value between 1 and 5.

- When your stomach signals true hunger, look for low energy density foods to fill it.

- Eat slowly to give your brain time to send the satiety signals back to your stomach.

- In choosing foods, consider the nutrient density of your choices to make sure you are giving your body the best advantages possible.

- If you still feel like eating when your stomach gives signals that it has reached satiety, discover other hungers you may be experiencing (see Parts 3, 4, and 5).

THE THIRD HUNGER

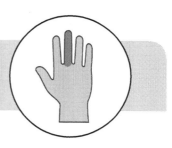

Middle Finger:
Hunger of Emotional Emptiness

- Look for "hunger" messages in poetry, literature and scriptures, and start noticing your own hunger-related emotions.

- Test your physical hunger by concentrating on the center of your abdomen and grow familiar with your body's *satiety* signals so you can be more aware of emotional needs.

- Track your hunger ratings, including both physical and emotional cues to eat, over three days or one week.

- Assess your stress level and read about stress management techniques.

- Modify recipes for your favorite comfort foods so they are healthier, reduce guilt, and fill you up physically with fewer calories.

- Experiment with new ways to fill your emotional emptiness such as intellectual stimulation, physical activity, or giving service.

THE FOURTH HUNGER

Ring Finger: Hunger for Stability

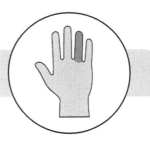

- Our bodies love habits and crave stability in routines, foods, activity patterns, and our surroundings.

- Food preferences originate early in life and can be heavily influenced by peers, advertising, and the media.

- Our habits become so ingrained they may feel like necessities.

- Habits are stronger than goals and often undermine our success in trying to eat healthier.

- High sugar and high fat foods create especially strong habits much like addictions.

- Food preferences and habits *can* be changed but the efforts to create healthy habits require significant attention.

- Use helpful resources from habit change research to assess and change your eating patterns.

- Consider your emotional needs and enlist help to support the transition as your changes will inevitably upset your body's craving for stability.

- Structure your personal environment to reinforce the changes you want to make.

THE FIFTH HUNGER

Pinky: Hunger for Novelty

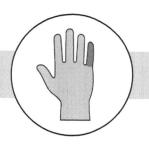

- Many people eat out of boredom or when they crave novelty, but the food fix is temporary and not what the body really needs.

- Our modern sedentary lifestyles have led to deficiencies in physical activity which harm our health and for which we need to find creative solutions.

- Our bones, joints, and circulatory systems crave movement especially given the sedentary lifestyles our modern conveniences provide.

- Moderate physical exercise can provide an energy boost and relieve fatigue.

- Any discussion of nutrition must include physical activity as a critical part of a person's nutritional status.

- Obsessions with weight loss instead of health lead to preoccupation with numbers on the scale. Our weight is a poor indicator of body composition.

- Healthy weight loss is slow and gradual and preserves lean body mass.

- One way to find the novelty your body hungers for is by taking an Activity Recess where you choose a physical activity that is fun and meets your own unique definition of recreation.

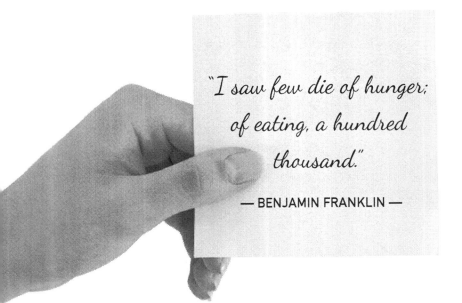

"I saw few die of hunger;
of eating, a hundred
thousand."

— BENJAMIN FRANKLIN —

FingerFOODS
Sample Recipes for each Hunger

Sample recipes from my book *The FIVE Diet* are provided here on the following tear-out pages for your convenience.

FingerFOODS for the First Hunger

In a rush to provide balanced meals for yourself or your family, to better control blood sugar levels? You don't have to resort to the drive-thru. In less than five minutes in the morning you can put together this hearty meal that will be ready for you at the end of your busy day.

Crock-Pot Vegetarian Chili in a Flash

2 16-oz cans black beans
1 16-oz can kidney beans
2 14.5-oz cans tomato sauce
2 Tbsp dried minced onions
2 1.25-oz pkgs chili seasoning
   (or your own seasoning mix made in advance)

Stir together all ingredients in Crock-Pot. Cook on low setting 8 to 12 hours.

Serve with optional toppings:
- Grated cheese
- Sour cream
- Fritos (corn chips)

Makes 10 1-cup servings

FingerFOODS for the Second Hunger

Help fill your empty stomach with this alternative to a traditional favorite. Veggie spaghetti has both lower energy density and higher nutrient density than spaghetti made with regular pasta.

This means you will be fuller on less food, and you will meet more of your body's nutritional needs at the same time.

Veggie Spaghetti has something for everyone—very low carb, gluten-free, high potassium . . . and the mild flavor fits in well with any traditional spaghetti sauce.

Veggie Spaghetti

1 medium spaghetti squash (cucurbita pepo)
4 cups marinara sauce, canned, bottled or made fresh
1 onion, chopped
1 cup mushrooms, diced
1 Tbsp olive oil
2 Tbsp grated parmesan cheese

Cut the squash in half and remove seeds.

Cook by roasting 30 to 40 minutes at 375° or boiling/steaming about 20 minutes. Best texture comes from being careful not to overcook. Squash is done when the strands separate easily with a fork.

Sauté onions and mushrooms in olive oil and stir in marinara sauce.

Serve over strands of squash. Top with parmesan cheese.

Makes 8 servings of 1 cup squash and ½ cup sauce

FingerFOODS for the Third Hunger

When you recognize when your hunger is really an emotional need, you can focus on addressing that issue. But we all can use a little comfort food once in a while. Here's one way to transform a traditional comfort food into a healthy addition to your meals. The healthier version will leave you more full and feeling less guilty!

Makeover Mashed Potatoes

Try a variety of vegetables, steamed and mashed, to replace or add to traditional mashed potatoes.

The following work well in mashed and creamy form:
- Cauliflower
- Butternut squash
- Parsnips
- Pumpkin

Peel and slice vegetables into 1-inch slices.

Bring to boil and simmer on low heat until tender, about 12 minutes. Drain, retaining liquid.

Mash in food processor or by hand. Add back some of the liquid to desired consistency. Lightly salt to taste.

TIP: mash an orange vegetable (cooked carrot or squash) in with white vegetables (cauliflower, potatoes or parsnips) for a buttery appearance that will fool your taste buds while being fat free!

FingerFOODS for the Fourth Hunger

Most of us tend to limit ourselves to the foods we have known and loved for years. One way to introduce yourself and your family to healthy new foods is to disguise them as old favorites.

Break a habit and learn to love tofu while you think you're eating good old scrambled eggs.

Tofu is worth introducing: low in calories, lactose-free, very high in complete protein, but free of cholesterol and saturated fats.

Tofu Scramble (you'll swear it's eggs)

1 14- to 16-oz block of firm tofu
½ cup chopped green onions
1 clove garlic, crushed (optional)
1 Tbsp olive oil
Salt and pepper

Sauté onion and garlic in oil. Drain tofu and mash with fork into sautéed vegetables, heat 5 minutes. Salt and pepper to taste. Best if served while warm.

Note: tofu will not overcook as eggs will if kept warm.

Optional toppings:
- Bacon or alternate
- Diced fresh tomatoes
- Grated cheese
- Your favorite omelet fillings

Makes 4 servings, each the size of 2 eggs

FingerFOODS for the Fifth Hunger

When you are hungering for novelty, don't fall for the media pressure to open a boring bag of chips or crackers. This colorful salsa is ultra-low-fat and packed with healthy fiber, protein and phytochemicals. Eat it with cucumber slices.

The bright colors and novel flavor combinations will energize you for a brisk walk with a friend.

Fiesta Black Bean Salsa

2 cups cooked black beans
   (1 16-oz can or cook from dry beans)
2 cups sweet corn: canned, frozen, or fresh
1 cup chopped green bell pepper
1 cup chopped red bell pepper
1 cup chopped yellow bell pepper
1 cup grated carrots
½ cup chopped cilantro (optional)
2 cups of your favorite salsa, bottled or made fresh

Drain and rinse beans and corn. Combine with chopped and grated vegetables. Add cilantro if desired. Will keep longer in refrigerator without added salsa, which can be added right before serving.

Can be used as a salad, dip, or side dish.

Index

"Our bodies are our gardens, to the which our wills are gardeners."

— WILLIAM SHAKESPEARE —

Index

Visit our web pages:

www.5hungers.com

www.letmereadit.com

16449273R00131

Made in the USA
Lexington, KY
24 July 2012